Safe Foods to Food Freedom

An Autistic Woman's Guide to Eating Disorder Recovery Through Accommodation, Not Assimilation

Jessamine Amelia Griffin

ISBN: 978-1-923646-23-0

First Edition, 2025

Disclaimer

This book is designed to provide information about eating disorder recovery for autistic individuals. It is sold with the understanding that the author and publisher are not engaged in rendering medical, psychological, or other professional services. If expert assistance or counseling is needed, the services of a competent professional should be sought.

The strategies and techniques described in this book represent the author's research and opinions based on current scientific literature. This book is not intended as a substitute for professional medical advice, diagnosis, or treatment. Always seek the advice of your physician, psychiatrist, therapist, registered dietitian, or other qualified health provider with any questions you may have regarding eating disorders, autism spectrum disorder, or any medical or mental health condition.

Eating disorders are serious mental health conditions that can be life-threatening. If you are experiencing a medical emergency, suicidal thoughts, or are in crisis, please contact emergency services immediately or call the National Eating Disorders Association Helpline at 1-800-931-2237, the National Suicide Prevention Lifeline at 988, or your local emergency number.

All case examples and personal stories included in this book are composite examples created for educational purposes, or details have been substantially altered to protect individual privacy. Any resemblance to specific individuals, living or deceased, is coincidental. Names including but not limited to Maria, James, Chen, Aisha, Diego, Priya, Marcus, Elena, Raj, Nicole, Jalila, Amina, Layla, Sofia, Isabella, Carlos, Miguel, Wei, Lin, and all other names used in examples are fictional identifiers and do not refer to actual persons.

While the author has made every effort to ensure the accuracy of information and references included in this book, neither the author nor the publisher assumes any responsibility for errors, inaccuracies, omissions, or

Preface

When I began researching the intersection of autism and eating disorders five years ago, I encountered a puzzle that wouldn't let me go. The clinical literature was clear: autistic women develop eating disorders at significantly higher rates than the general population. Between 20 and 35% of women with anorexia nervosa meet diagnostic criteria for autism. The co-occurrence isn't coincidental—it's structural. Yet when I looked for resources that autistic women could actually use to recover, I found almost nothing.

There were clinical texts for professionals. A handful of memoirs. But no practical, comprehensive guide that explained why standard eating disorder treatment so often fails autistic individuals and what actually works instead. That gap—between knowing the problem exists and providing accessible solutions—is why this book exists.

I'm a researcher who has spent years studying eating disorders, autism spectrum disorders, and the specific challenges that emerge when these conditions intersect. My work has taken me through clinical literature, treatment center observations, interviews with autistic women who've survived eating disorders, and consultations with the few clinicians who specialize in this intersection. What I found, consistently, was a disconnect. The research exists. Clinicians like Dr. Kate Tchanturia have developed adapted treatment protocols. The PEACE Pathway demonstrates that autism-informed approaches work. But this knowledge remains largely trapped in academic journals and specialized treatment centers.

Meanwhile, autistic women sit in eating disorder treatment programs designed for neurotypical brains, being told to eat intuitively when they can't feel hunger, to be flexible when their neurology requires structure, to process emotions they can't name, and to tolerate sensory environments that overwhelm them. They're labeled treatment-resistant, oppositional, or unmotivated when they struggle with approaches that fundamentally don't match their neurology.

Then they're discharged, still struggling, still without the accommodations they actually need.

This isn't theoretical for me. Through my research, I've met too many women who spent years cycling through treatment programs that couldn't help them—not because their eating disorders were more severe, but because their autism was never properly addressed. I've read countless stories in online communities of autistic women who gave up on recovery because every approach they tried demanded they stop being autistic while recovering from their eating disorder. Stop needing routine. Stop being sensitive to sensory input. Stop thinking in patterns. Just be normal, and recovery will follow.

Except it doesn't work that way.

Recovery is possible for autistic women with eating disorders. But it requires different approaches. It requires understanding that your need for structure isn't eating disorder rigidity—it's autism accommodation. That your sensory food preferences aren't all restriction—some are genuine neurological differences. That your difficulty with interoception isn't resistance—it's how your nervous system processes internal signals. That your alexithymia isn't emotional avoidance—it's a real challenge in identifying feelings that requires adapted strategies.

This book brings together what research knows about autism and eating disorders with what autistic women actually need: practical strategies that work with your neurology instead of against it. Every chapter addresses a specific aspect of recovery adapted for autistic brains. The approaches here aren't my invention—they're drawn from emerging clinical protocols, autism research, neurodiversity frameworks, and the lived experience of autistic women who've found recovery paths that actually sustained.

You'll notice this book doesn't read like a typical self-help book. That's intentional. The voice is direct, sometimes technical, always straightforward. Autistic readers consistently tell me they prefer clear information without excessive emotional language or presumptuous statements about their experiences. I've tried to honor that preference while maintaining warmth and genuine support.

The book is structured to build progressively. Early chapters establish why standard treatment fails and what you need instead. Middle chapters provide specific strategies for sensory issues, interoception, rigid thinking, and emotional regulation. Final chapters address long-term recovery maintenance and living fully as an autistic person free from eating disorder control. Each chapter includes research citations because you deserve to know where information comes from and verify it yourself if desired. Case examples throughout illustrate concepts, but they're composites created for educational purposes, not real individuals.

A note about language: I use identity-first language ("autistic person") rather than person-first language ("person with autism") because most autistic self-advocates prefer this construction. Autism isn't something you have—it's part of who you are. Similarly, I often use "eating disorder" as a noun rather than always saying "person with an eating disorder" because cumbersome language serves no one. If different terminology works better for you, mentally substitute as you read.

This book assumes you're either autistic yourself or strongly suspect you might be. If you're unsure about your autism, the content will still help—many women discover their autism only after eating disorder treatment repeatedly fails. The strategies here work regardless of official diagnosis because they address real neurological differences, not arbitrary labels.

What this book won't do: cure your autism (autism isn't an illness), make you neurotypical (impossible and undesirable), promise you'll love all foods (sensory preferences are real), or guarantee you'll eat "normally" (normal is overrated and poorly defined). What this book will do: help you eat consistently and adequately as the autistic person you are, break free from eating disorder control, build accommodations that support sustained recovery, and create a life worth nourishing.

I wrote this book because autistic women deserve recovery resources designed for their neurology, not despite it. You deserve treatment that accommodates your sensory processing, supports your need for structure, works with your interoception difficulties, and respects your autistic identity. You deserve to recover without becoming someone else.

You don't need to read this book linearly. Skip to chapters addressing your most pressing challenges. Return to sections as you need them. Use what works, adapt what doesn't, and trust yourself to know what your recovery requires. Your autism gives you particular strengths—pattern recognition, attention to detail, systematic thinking—that can support recovery when properly channeled. The same neurology that complicates eating can also facilitate sustained change when you have the right approaches.

Recovery is possible. Not despite your autism, but with it.
.Jessamine Amelia Griffin

Table of Contents

Chapter 1.0: Understanding Autism and Eating Disorders

You've probably heard the statistics about eating disorders. You know they're dangerous. You know they affect millions of people. But here's what most people don't know: if you're an autistic woman, your risk isn't just higher—it's three times higher than your neurotypical peers (Westwood & Tchanturia, 2017). And the treatment approach that works for everyone else? It often doesn't work for you. Not because you're doing it wrong, but because the treatment itself wasn't designed with your autistic brain in mind.

This chapter explores why autism and eating disorders so often collide, how this intersection gets misunderstood by clinicians, and what you need to know to make sense of your own experience. Whether you've been diagnosed with anorexia, bulimia, ARFID, or you're still trying to figure out what's going on with food, understanding how your autism influences your eating patterns changes everything.

1.1 The Triple Risk Factor

Let's start with the numbers, because they're striking. Research consistently shows that 20-30% of people in treatment for anorexia nervosa are autistic (Westwood & Tchanturia, 2017). Think about that. In a room of ten people receiving eating disorder treatment, two or three are on the autism spectrum. Compare that to the general population, where only about 1% of women are autistic (Loomes et al., 2017). The math is clear: something about being autistic dramatically increases eating disorder risk.

But why? The answer isn't simple, and it's not just one thing. Autistic women face a perfect storm of risk factors that neurotypical women don't encounter. First, there's the sensory processing differences. Your brain might experience certain food textures as genuinely unbearable—not just disliked, but physically distressing

(Kinnaird et al., 2019). Second, autistic brains tend toward pattern-based thinking and rule-following. When diet culture tells you to follow rigid food rules, your brain latches onto those rules with an intensity that can quickly spiral into restriction (Brede et al., 2020). Third, many autistic people struggle with interoception—the ability to sense internal body signals like hunger and fullness. When you can't reliably feel when you're hungry, establishing normal eating patterns becomes genuinely difficult (Kinnaird et al., 2019).

Add to this the chronic stress of living in a world not designed for autistic brains. The constant masking, the social exhaustion, the sensory overload. Food becomes one of the few things you can control when everything else feels chaotic. One study found that autistic women with anorexia often developed eating disorders as a way to manage overwhelming anxiety and emotional dysregulation (Brede et al., 2020). The eating disorder wasn't primarily about wanting to be thin—it was about finding something predictable and controllable in an unpredictable world.

1.2 When Your Eating Disorder Gets Diagnosed First

Here's a pattern that shows up over and over in research and clinical practice: an autistic woman develops an eating disorder in her teens or twenties, gets diagnosed and treated for the eating disorder, but her autism goes completely unrecognized. Sometimes for years. Sometimes for decades.

The average age gap is startling. In one study, autistic women were diagnosed with anorexia at an average age of 17, but didn't receive their autism diagnosis until age 29—a full 12 years later (Babb et al., 2021). Twelve years of treatment that didn't account for their autism. Twelve years of feeling like something was wrong with them because standard eating disorder treatment wasn't working the way it should.

Why does this happen? Several reasons. First, eating disorder symptoms can mask autism symptoms. When you're severely underweight and malnourished, you might show social withdrawal, rigid thinking, and sensory sensitivities—but clinicians attribute these to starvation, not autism (Westwood et al., 2016). They're waiting for you to recover from the eating disorder to see your "real" personality. Except those traits don't go away with weight restoration, because they were autism traits all along.

Second, diagnostic bias plays a huge role. Clinicians have been trained to look for autism primarily in boys and men. The "classic" autism presentation—the one most professionals learned about—doesn't match how autism presents in many women. Autistic women often develop sophisticated masking strategies, copying social behaviors from peers, and hiding their struggles (Bargiela et al., 2016). You might make eye contact, have friendships, and seem socially competent to outsiders. But internally, you're exhausted from the constant effort of appearing neurotypical.

Third, when you're already in eating disorder treatment, clinicians develop what's called "diagnostic overshadowing." They see everything through the eating disorder lens. Your need for routine? That's the anorexia making you rigid. Your sensory issues with food? That's restrictive eating. Your social difficulties? That's the eating disorder isolating you. Nobody stops to ask: what if these traits existed before the eating disorder and will persist after recovery?

1.3 How Autism Traits Fuel Disordered Eating

Understanding the specific autism traits that contribute to eating disorders helps you recognize patterns in your own experience. These aren't excuses—they're explanations that can guide more effective recovery strategies.

Sensory sensitivities affect up to 90% of autistic people (Tomchek & Dunn, 2007). For many autistic women, certain food textures trigger genuine disgust or even panic. Mushy foods, slimy foods, foods with unexpected textures—these aren't just preferences. Your sensory system processes them as threats. When you're already anxious about eating, adding foods that trigger sensory distress becomes nearly impossible. Over time, your safe food list shrinks. You're not being "picky"—your nervous system is genuinely overwhelmed.

Alexithymia—difficulty identifying and describing emotions—affects about 50% of autistic adults (Bird & Cook, 2013). When you can't easily distinguish between emotional discomfort and physical sensations, it becomes hard to know when you're actually hungry versus anxious, sad, or overwhelmed. Many autistic women report that they don't feel hunger cues clearly, or they confuse anxiety symptoms with fullness. This makes intuitive eating—the approach recommended in most eating disorder recovery programs—extremely challenging.

Need for routine and sameness is a core autism trait. Routines feel safe. Predictability reduces anxiety. But eating disorders thrive on rigid routines. When diet culture introduces rules about "good" and "bad" foods, meal timing, and eating rituals, autistic brains can lock onto these rules with intense focus. What starts as a diet becomes an unbreakable routine. Research shows that autistic individuals with eating disorders demonstrate significantly higher cognitive rigidity compared to non-autistic people with eating disorders (Westwood et al., 2016). Your brain's natural inclination toward pattern-based thinking amplifies eating disorder behaviors.

Executive function challenges affect planning, organization, and task initiation. Meal planning requires deciding what to eat, shopping for ingredients, preparing food, and timing meals appropriately. For many autistic people, this entire sequence feels overwhelming. It's easier to eat the same thing repeatedly, skip meals due to decision fatigue, or rely on others to manage food. These patterns can evolve into or maintain eating disorder behaviors.

1.4 ARFID or Anorexia

Here's where diagnostic confusion becomes critical. Avoidant/Restrictive Food Intake Disorder (ARFID) was added to the DSM-5 in 2013, and it's particularly relevant for autistic individuals. ARFID involves restricted eating that causes significant weight loss or nutritional deficiency, but—and this is key—it's not driven by concerns about weight or body image (American Psychiatric Association, 2013).

For autistic people, food avoidance often stems from sensory sensitivities, lack of interest in eating, or fear of adverse consequences like choking or vomiting. Research shows that approximately 44% of children and adolescents with ARFID are autistic (Nicely et al., 2014). That's nearly half. Yet many autistic women with sensory-based food restriction get diagnosed with anorexia nervosa instead, because their restricted eating causes low body weight.

Why does the distinction matter? Treatment differs significantly. Anorexia treatment focuses heavily on challenging beliefs about body image, weight, and appearance. Cognitive-behavioral therapy for anorexia targets thoughts like "I'm fat" or "eating will make me gain too much weight." But if you have ARFID, those aren't your thoughts. You're avoiding foods because they trigger sensory distress, not because you're afraid of weight gain. Being pushed through body image work when that's not your issue wastes time and creates frustration.

Consider Elena, a 28-year-old autistic woman diagnosed with anorexia at age 16. She spent over a decade in various eating disorder programs, consistently told her treatment wasn't working because she "wasn't trying hard enough" to challenge her distorted body image. The problem? Elena didn't have distorted body image. She could look in a mirror and accurately assess her body. What she couldn't do was eat foods with certain textures without gagging. She couldn't eat in noisy cafeterias without becoming overwhelmed. She couldn't meal plan without feeling paralyzed by too many choices. After finally receiving an autism assessment and ARFID diagnosis at age 27, Elena's treatment shifted to sensory integration strategies, routine establishment, and gradual texture exposure. Within six months, she made more progress than she had in the previous ten years.

That said, the picture isn't always clear-cut. Some autistic women do develop anorexia with body image concerns. Others have a mixed presentation—sensory issues plus weight concerns. Recent research suggests that for autistic women with restrictive eating, both ARFID and anorexia features may be present simultaneously (Brede et al., 2020). The point isn't to fit neatly into one box or another. The point is ensuring your treatment addresses the actual drivers of your eating disorder, not assumed drivers based on stereotypes.

1.5 Why Standard Treatment Fails

Standard eating disorder treatment follows evidence-based protocols developed through research on primarily non-autistic populations. These treatments work well for many people. But they often fail for autistic women. Let's look at why.

Group therapy is a cornerstone of many eating disorder programs. Patients sit in groups, sharing experiences and supporting each other. For many people, this is healing. For autistic women, it can be torture. The social demands, the unpredictable conversations, the emotional intensity, the fluorescent lights, the inability to leave when overstimulated—all of these create barriers to engagement (Babb et al., 2021). You're supposed to focus on recovery, but you're spending all your energy managing sensory overload and social exhaustion.

Exposure-based interventions in eating disorder treatment involve eating fear foods in challenging environments. You might be asked to eat pizza in a restaurant, have dessert at a party, or order food spontaneously without planning. These exposures are designed to challenge anxious avoidance. But for autistic people, some avoidance is adaptive. Eating in noisy, chaotic environments genuinely impairs your ability to process internal signals. The stress of unpredictability isn't irrational—your nervous system requires more predictability to function optimally. When treatment pushes you to "face your fears" without distinguishing between eating disorder anxiety and autism-related stress, it can be retraumatizing rather than therapeutic.

Intuitive eating approaches tell you to "listen to your body" and "eat when you're hungry." This advice assumes you can reliably detect hunger and fullness signals. If you have interoception difficulties, this approach fails immediately. You're told to trust your body's signals when your body's signals are unclear or absent. Rather than feeling empowered, you feel like you're failing at something that should be natural.

Emphasis on flexibility runs through eating disorder treatment. You're encouraged to eat spontaneously, vary your foods, challenge rigid rules. But cognitive flexibility is specifically challenging for autistic brains (Westwood et al., 2016). Being told to "just be more flexible" isn't helpful—it's like telling someone with depression to "just be happier." The advice isn't wrong exactly, but without strategies that account for how your brain actually works, it's useless.

A study examining autistic women's experiences of eating disorder services found three major themes: misunderstanding of autism, one-size-fits-all treatment, and poor accessibility (Babb et al., 2021). Healthcare professionals acknowledged that standard protocols didn't work well for autistic patients, but few had training in adapting treatment appropriately. The result? Autistic women stay in treatment longer, have worse outcomes, and are more likely to be readmitted after discharge compared to non-autistic women with eating disorders (Kinnaird et al., 2017).

1.6 Autism Versus Severe Anorexia

Here's a critical distinction that gets confused constantly: some behaviors that look like severe eating disorder symptoms are actually autism traits. When you're in acute stages of anorexia—severely underweight and malnourished—you might show social withdrawal, rigid thinking, restricted interests, repetitive behaviors, and sensory sensitivities. These are also autism traits.

Clinicians often assume these behaviors will resolve with nutritional rehabilitation and weight restoration. For non-autistic patients, they often do. The brain returns to normal functioning, and the person becomes more flexible, more social, more able to tolerate uncertainty. But for autistic women, these traits persist after weight restoration because they were there all along (Bentz et al., 2017).

This creates a frustrating dynamic. You complete residential treatment, restore weight, and your treatment team expects you to be "better." But you still need routine. You still find social situations exhausting. You still have sensory sensitivities. Your team might interpret this as treatment resistance or insufficient recovery, when actually, you're autistic. The traits they're seeing aren't eating disorder symptoms—they're autism. They're part of who you are, not part of what you need to cure.

Research using rigorous diagnostic tools confirms this. Even after recovery from anorexia, approximately 25% of women continue to meet full diagnostic criteria for autism (Westwood et al., 2017). These aren't pseudo-autistic traits created by starvation. They're genuine autism that was present before the eating disorder and persists after.

Understanding this distinction matters for treatment planning. If your clinician thinks your need for routine is eating disorder rigidity, they'll push you to be more spontaneous. But if it's autism-related need for predictability, pushing flexibility without support will increase your distress rather than helping recovery. You need strategies that honor your neurological differences while still supporting eating disorder recovery.

1.7 The Twenty to Thirty Percent

Let's return to that statistic: 20-30% of people with anorexia nervosa are autistic (Westwood & Tchanturia, 2017). What does this actually mean for you?

First, you're not alone. If you're an autistic woman struggling with an eating disorder, you're part of a significant population. Your experience isn't strange or unusual—it's a well-documented pattern that researchers and clinicians are finally starting to understand.

Second, this prevalence rate is high enough that it should change treatment practices. When roughly one-quarter of eating disorder patients are autistic, "standard" treatment should include autism accommodations as routine practice, not special exceptions. The PEACE Pathway, developed at the Maudsley Hospital in London, is one of the first eating disorder treatment programs specifically designed for autistic individuals (Tchanturia et al., 2020). It includes sensory-friendly environments, autism psychoeducation, accommodations for executive function challenges, and staff training in autism awareness. Early results show promising outcomes.

Third, this statistic highlights the urgent need for better autism screening in eating disorder settings. A study examining eating disorder professionals' ability to identify autism found that they successfully recognized autism in 17.5% of previously undiagnosed adolescent and young adult females entering treatment (Parsons et al., 2023). That's good—but it also means some autistic patients are still being missed. Every eating disorder assessment should include autism screening, particularly for women and girls.

1.8 What This Means for You

Understanding the autism-eating disorder connection isn't about creating excuses or feeling doomed. It's about accurate understanding that leads to effective strategies.

If you're autistic and struggling with disordered eating, you need treatment that accounts for both conditions. That means sensory accommodations, structured routines that support recovery rather than restriction, strategies for improving interoception, and support for executive function challenges. It means clinicians who understand that your need for sameness isn't something to simply "break through," but something to work with strategically.

Recovery is absolutely possible for autistic women with eating disorders. But recovery might look different than it does for neurotypical people. Your version of recovery might include keeping some routines, continuing to avoid certain textures that genuinely distress you, and eating in structured ways that work with your brain rather than against it. That's not failed recovery—that's autism-affirming recovery.

The research is clear: when eating disorder treatment is adapted to meet the specific needs of autistic individuals, outcomes improve significantly (Tchanturia et al., 2021). The problem hasn't been that autistic people can't recover. The problem has been that treatment hasn't been adapted appropriately.

You deserve treatment that sees all of you—your autism and your eating disorder. Understanding how these conditions intersect in your life is the first step toward finding approaches that actually work.

Chapter 2.0: The Autistic Eating Experience

If one more person tells you you're "just picky," you might scream. But here's the truth: what looks like pickiness from the outside is often something completely different on the inside. Your relationship with food has layers that most people don't experience. Sensory processing differences, difficulties sensing internal body signals, executive function challenges, and the sheer exhaustion of navigating food in a world that doesn't understand autism—all of these shape how you eat.

This chapter explores the specific ways autism affects eating, separate from eating disorder diagnosis. Understanding your autistic eating experience helps you distinguish between what's autism, what's eating disorder, and what's the complicated overlap between the two. That clarity matters. It's the foundation for recovery strategies that actually work with your brain instead of fighting against it.

2.1 Safe Foods and Sensory Processing

Let's talk about safe foods. You probably have a mental list—maybe short, maybe a bit longer—of foods you can reliably eat without distress. These aren't just foods you prefer. They're foods your nervous system tolerates. Everything else exists on a spectrum from "maybe if I have to" to "absolutely not possible."

The sensory experience of eating involves more systems than most people realize. Taste, obviously. But also texture, temperature, smell, visual appearance, and even the sound food makes when you chew it. For autistic individuals, one or more of these sensory channels might process information differently, often more intensely (Cermak et al., 2010).

Texture is the big one for many autistic people. Certain textures—slimy, mushy, grainy, or foods with mixed textures—can trigger genuine disgust responses. This isn't preference. It's not being stubborn. Research using brain imaging shows that for individuals with sensory processing differences, aversive textures activate threat-detection areas of the brain (Tavassoli et al., 2012). Your brain literally processes these textures as dangerous.

Consider Marcus, a 32-year-old autistic man recovering from what was diagnosed as anorexia but later recognized as ARFID. Marcus could eat crackers, plain pasta, chicken nuggets, and apple slices. That was it. Treatment teams pushed him to expand his foods, bringing in pizzas with melted cheese, casseroles with mixed textures, and smoothies. Marcus would gag, sometimes vomit, and refuse to try again. Clinicians interpreted this as eating disorder behavior—avoidance motivated by fear of calories or weight gain. But Marcus wasn't afraid of gaining weight. He was terrified of the sensory experience itself. The stringy, stretchy texture of melted cheese made his skin crawl. Mixed textures where he couldn't predict what each bite would feel like triggered panic. Once treatment shifted to gradual texture exposure using behavioral strategies from occupational therapy, Marcus made steady progress. Six months later, he was eating 30 different foods—not by forcing himself through distress, but by slowly building tolerance through supported exposure.

Safe foods often share characteristics: predictable texture, familiar taste, consistent appearance. You know exactly what each bite will be like. There's comfort in that predictability. When life feels overwhelming and unpredictable, safe foods offer something you can count on.

But here's where it gets complicated: eating disorder behaviors can co-opt sensory sensitivities. Maybe you genuinely dislike certain textures. But maybe you've also started avoiding foods because they're "too caloric" or "too messy" or "too scary" for eating disorder reasons. Distinguishing genuine sensory avoidance from eating disorder avoidance requires honest reflection. Does the food trigger physical disgust responses? Or does it trigger anxiety about eating it? Sometimes it's both. That's okay. You can work with both.

2.2 When Your Body Doesn't Send Clear Signals

Interoception is your ability to sense internal body signals: hunger, fullness, thirst, need to use the bathroom, heart rate, breathing, temperature, pain. Most people process these signals automatically. Autistic individuals often don't (Garfinkel et al., 2016).

Poor interoception doesn't mean you never feel hunger. It means hunger signals might be:

- Weak or subtle, easy to miss
- Delayed, showing up hours after your body actually needed food
- Confused with other sensations (anxiety, stomach discomfort, fatigue)
- Completely absent until you're extremely hungry and it hits suddenly
- Present but not recognizable as hunger

Research shows that autistic adults score significantly lower on interoception awareness measures compared to non-autistic adults (Garfinkel et al., 2016). About 70% of autistic individuals report difficulties with interoception (DuBois et al., 2016). That's a huge majority. If you struggle to know when you're hungry or full, you're not broken or doing something wrong. Your nervous system processes these signals differently.

When you can't rely on hunger cues, eating becomes a cognitive task rather than an intuitive response. You have to think about when to eat, plan meals, set reminders. This works fine until you're stressed, overwhelmed, or dealing with executive function challenges. Then meals get skipped. Not because you're restricting intentionally, but because you genuinely forgot to eat or didn't notice you needed food.

Now add an eating disorder to this picture. Many eating disorders involve deliberately ignoring or suppressing hunger cues. But if your hunger cues were already unclear, the eating disorder makes everything worse. You might convince yourself you're not hungry when your body desperately needs nutrition, but you genuinely can't tell the difference between "not hungry" and "suppressing hunger."

Recovery programs often emphasize "listening to your body" and eating intuitively. This advice assumes reliable interoception. Without it, the advice is useless. You need structured eating patterns—planned meals and snacks at regular times—to ensure adequate nutrition regardless of what your body signals are or aren't telling you.

Priya, a 26-year-old autistic woman in recovery from anorexia, describes it this way: "Everyone kept saying 'eat when you're hungry, stop when you're full.' But I never felt hungry. Or I'd suddenly feel starving after not eating all day, then eat too much and feel sick. Or I'd feel something uncomfortable in my stomach and couldn't tell if it was hunger, anxiety, or fullness. I spent hours trying to 'listen to my body' when my body wasn't speaking a language I could understand."

Priya's breakthrough came when her dietitian stopped pushing intuitive eating and instead created a structured meal plan. Three meals, two snacks, specific times. Priya didn't have to figure out if she was hungry. She just had to follow the schedule. Within weeks, her nutrition stabilized. After several months of consistent eating, her interoception improved slightly—she started noticing some hunger signals. But the structure remained necessary. For Priya, eating needed external scaffolding because internal signals weren't reliable enough.

2.3 Executive Function and Meal Planning Paralysis

Executive function refers to cognitive processes that help you plan, organize, initiate tasks, manage time, and follow through on goals. Many autistic individuals experience executive function challenges

(Demetriou et al., 2018). When it comes to eating, executive function affects every step:

Deciding what to eat requires processing multiple factors: what foods you have available, what sounds appealing, what you're in the mood for, what's nutritionally appropriate, how much time you have to prepare it. For many autistic people, this decision tree becomes overwhelming. Too many variables. Too many possibilities. Decision paralysis sets in.

Shopping for food involves planning a shopping list, navigating a crowded, sensory-intense store, making hundreds of micro-decisions, and managing time and budget. Executive function challenges make each step harder.

Preparing food requires sequencing multiple steps, managing timing, monitoring multiple elements simultaneously (something on the stove, something in the oven, something that needs chopping), and adapting when things don't go as planned. When executive function is impaired, cooking becomes genuinely difficult.

Cleaning up adds another layer of steps after you're already exhausted from the previous stages.

No wonder many autistic people eat the same foods repeatedly or rely on convenience foods. It's not laziness. It's executive function conservation. When you have limited cognitive resources, spending them on elaborate meal planning and preparation doesn't make sense.

But eating disorders complicate this further. Eating disorder rules add more decision points. "Is this food safe?" "How many calories?" "When did I last eat?" "Will this make me gain weight?" "What will people think if I eat this?" Each additional rule compounds the executive function load. Many autistic women with eating disorders describe food decisions becoming so overwhelming that they just... don't eat. It's not purposeful restriction. It's executive function shutdown.

Chen, a 24-year-old autistic graduate student, developed bulimia during her first year of graduate school. Between research demands, teaching responsibilities, and coursework, Chen's executive function was maxed out. Meal planning felt impossible. She'd stand in front of the refrigerator for ten minutes, unable to decide what to eat. Eventually she'd eat nothing, or grab something quick, or binge on whatever was immediately accessible, then purge because the binge felt out of control.

Recovery involved radical simplification. Chen's therapist helped her create a rotation of five breakfast options, five lunch options, and five dinner options. Same foods every week. No decisions. Monday breakfast was always overnight oats. Tuesday lunch was always a turkey sandwich. This structure eliminated decision-making and reduced executive function demands. Within that structure, Chen's eating stabilized. Was it exciting? No. Did it work? Yes.

2.4 The Rigidity Trap

Autistic brains tend toward pattern-based thinking. You notice patterns, create rules, and follow those rules consistently. This can be a strength—it helps with systematic thinking, attention to detail, and expertise in specific areas. But when diet culture enters your life with its endless rules about food, your brain can latch onto those rules with intensity that quickly becomes harmful.

"Don't eat after 8 PM." "No carbs at breakfast." "Protein at every meal." "No snacking between meals." "Only eat when truly hungry." Diet culture presents these as health rules. Your brain, wired for pattern recognition and rule-following, treats them as absolute laws. Breaking a rule creates significant anxiety. Following rules creates relief. This is how eating disorders develop and maintain themselves in many autistic people—not primarily through body image distortion, but through rigid adherence to food rules (Westwood et al., 2016).

Research on cognitive inflexibility in autism and eating disorders shows that autistic individuals with anorexia demonstrate significantly more rigid thinking patterns than non-autistic individuals with anorexia (Westwood et al., 2016). Your brain's natural preference for rules and routines amplifies eating disorder behaviors.

Here's what makes it especially difficult: some routine around eating is adaptive for autistic people. Structure helps. Predictability reduces anxiety. The challenge is distinguishing between helpful routine and harmful rigidity. Helpful routine might be eating at consistent times each day. Harmful rigidity is refusing to eat if the meal is ten minutes late or if your safe food isn't available.

Recovery requires developing flexibility while maintaining enough structure to support your autistic needs. This balance is tricky. You need some flexibility—enough that you can eat in imperfect circumstances, with some variation in foods and timing. But you also need structure—enough that executive function demands don't become overwhelming and anxiety stays manageable.

2.5 Food as Emotional Control

Emotional regulation—the ability to manage emotional intensity and respond appropriately to feelings—is challenging for many autistic people (Mazefsky et al., 2013). Emotions can feel overwhelming, intense, and difficult to modulate. When you add the fact that many autistic individuals struggle to identify what emotion they're feeling (alexithymia), managing emotions becomes genuinely difficult.

Food enters this picture as one of the few things you can control. Your emotions might feel chaotic. Social situations might be unpredictable. Sensory environments might be overwhelming. But food? You can control food. What you eat, when you eat, how much you eat—these are within your power.

For some autistic women, restriction becomes a way to create calm. When everything feels too much, not eating quiets the intensity.

Your body shuts down, energy decreases, and overwhelming emotions dull. This isn't healthy, but it works as a short-term coping strategy. Research shows that many autistic women report using eating disorder behaviors specifically to manage emotional dysregulation rather than to change their body shape (Brede et al., 2020).

For others, binge eating serves a similar function. When emotions become unbearable, eating provides temporary relief. Food can be soothing, numbing, distracting. It's something to do with your hands and mouth that isn't screaming or crying or hurting yourself.

Aisha, a 29-year-old autistic woman, described her binge-purge cycle this way: "When I get overwhelmed—too much noise, too much social interaction, too many demands—I feel like I'm going to explode. Everything inside me is screaming. Binge eating is the only thing that makes it stop. For 20 minutes while I'm eating, I don't feel anything except the sensation of chewing and swallowing. It's the only relief I can find. Then I purge because I panic about what I just ate. I know it's not healthy. But I don't have other ways to handle the emotional intensity."

Aisha's recovery involved two parallel tracks. First, addressing the eating disorder behaviors—establishing regular eating patterns, challenging binge-purge cycles, processing shame around eating. Second, developing alternative emotion regulation strategies specific to autistic nervous systems: sensory tools (weighted blanket, fidget objects, noise-canceling headphones), movement breaks, special interest engagement, and structured downtime after overwhelming experiences.

The point isn't that food control is good. It's understanding why food became your coping mechanism. When you're autistic, navigating emotions is harder than most clinicians recognize. Food offers concrete, controllable, immediate relief. Letting go of eating disorder behaviors means finding alternative strategies that work with your autistic neurology.

2.6 Social Eating and Masking Exhaustion

Eating is intensely social in most cultures. Meals bring people together. Food is served at celebrations, meetings, dates, family gatherings. For autistic people, social eating creates multiple layers of challenge.

First, the social demands themselves. Making conversation, maintaining appropriate eye contact, reading social cues, knowing when to speak and when to listen, understanding jokes or sarcasm—all of these require conscious effort for many autistic people. This is masking: working hard to appear neurotypical in social situations (Bargiela et al., 2016). Masking is exhausting. It requires constant monitoring of your behavior and active suppression of autistic traits.

Now add eating to the social situation. You're managing social interaction while also coordinating the physical act of eating: cutting food, bringing it to your mouth, chewing quietly, not spilling, timing bites appropriately so you're not eating while someone asks you a question. If you have any sensory sensitivities, the restaurant environment adds more challenge: bright lights, loud conversations, strong smells, crowded seating.

Many autistic women report that they can either eat or socialize, but not both simultaneously. The cognitive load is too high. So they push food around their plate, take tiny bites, or avoid eating entirely until they're alone. From the outside, this looks like eating disorder behavior. And sometimes it becomes eating disorder behavior—patterns established during social eating situations generalize to eating alone as well.

Research on social eating in autism shows that social meal contexts significantly increase anxiety and reduce food intake compared to eating alone (Lucarelli et al., 2017). This isn't eating disorder pathology. It's autism affecting eating in social contexts.

Isabella, a 35-year-old autistic woman, realized that most of her eating disorder behaviors started in social situations. She'd go out to dinner with friends and be unable to eat because she was working so hard to appear engaged, interested, and socially appropriate. She'd come home exhausted and starving but too tired to prepare food. Eventually, she started avoiding social meals entirely. Friends thought she was antisocial or didn't like them. Actually, Isabella was protecting herself from overwhelming experiences.

Recovery involved Isabella learning to set boundaries around social eating. She started meeting friends for coffee after meals instead of during meals. When she did eat with others, she chose quiet restaurants, arrived early to adjust to the environment, and gave herself permission to focus more on eating than conversation. She also stopped forcing herself to attend every social eating event. Sometimes staying home and eating alone was the right choice. This wasn't avoidance—it was appropriate accommodation.

2.7 Identifying Your Personal Intersections

Your autism and your eating disorder interact in ways specific to you. Understanding your personal pattern requires honest reflection. Here are questions to consider:

About sensory experiences:

- Which food textures genuinely distress you versus which do you avoid for eating disorder reasons?
- Do you avoid foods because of how they feel in your mouth, or because of their caloric content?
- Are there foods you used to enjoy that you now avoid? What changed?

About interoception:

- Can you reliably identify hunger? How do you know you're hungry?
- Can you distinguish between physical hunger, anxiety, and other uncomfortable sensations?

- Do you sometimes realize hours later that you forgot to eat? What was happening when you forgot?

About executive function:

- Does meal planning feel overwhelming? Which specific steps are hardest?
- Do you eat the same foods repeatedly because you genuinely prefer them, or because deciding what to eat feels impossible?
- How much cognitive energy does food preparation require for you?

About rigidity:

- Which eating rules do you follow? Where did they come from?
- What happens emotionally when you can't follow your food rules?
- Which routines around eating help you versus which ones restrict you?

About emotional regulation:

- Do you use food behaviors (restricting, bingeing, purging) to manage emotions?
- Which emotions are hardest for you to handle?
- What happens emotionally right before engaging in eating disorder behaviors?

About social eating:

- Do you eat differently alone versus with others?
- What specifically is hard about eating in social situations?
- Do you avoid social events because of the eating component?

There are no wrong answers. The goal is clarity. Understanding where your autism ends and your eating disorder begins helps you develop targeted strategies. Some patterns need to change completely. Others need accommodation and support rather than elimination. Only you can determine which is which, though working with knowledgeable professionals helps.

2.8 Moving Forward with Clarity

Understanding your autistic eating experience doesn't solve everything, but it provides crucial foundation. You're not defective or uniquely difficult to treat. You're autistic, and autism affects eating in predictable, well-documented ways.

Recovery strategies that work for non-autistic people often need adaptation for autistic brains. You might need more structure, not less. More predictability, not more flexibility. Sensory accommodations, not just exposure. Explicit teaching of interoception skills, not assumptions that you'll "just know" when you're hungry. Support for executive function, not judgments about laziness.

Your version of recovery will include accommodating your autism while addressing eating disorder behaviors. This means developing flexibility where it helps (being able to eat imperfect meals, tolerating some unpredictability, expanding foods gradually) while maintaining structure where it supports you (regular meal times, consistent routines, sensory-friendly eating environments).

The following chapters provide specific strategies for building this recovery approach. You'll learn how to work with your sensory system instead of fighting it, how to improve interoception, how to manage exccutive function demands, how to develop appropriate flexibility, and how to handle emotions without using food. All of these strategies are designed specifically for autistic brains, not adapted from approaches designed for neurotypical people.

Understanding is the first step. Action comes next. And action, informed by accurate understanding of your autistic neurology, creates real, sustainable recovery.

Chapter 3.0: Rewriting the Recovery Rules

You tried treatment. Maybe multiple times. Residential programs, intensive outpatient, therapy, dietitians. You followed the rules, showed up to groups, ate the meal plan. But something fundamental wasn't working. The treatment that helped your roommate or your friend left you feeling more broken, not less. Here's what nobody told you: standard eating disorder treatment wasn't designed for autistic brains. The approaches that work for neurotypical people often fail for autistic women—not because you're treatment-resistant, but because the treatment itself needs adaptation.

This chapter examines why traditional eating disorder interventions so often miss the mark for autistic individuals and what actually needs to happen instead. Understanding where treatment went wrong helps you advocate for what you actually need.

3.1 The Weight Obsession Problem

Standard eating disorder treatment centers weight as the primary metric of recovery. Weigh-ins happen weekly, sometimes daily. Treatment teams track BMI, calculate target weights, and tie privileges to weight gain. The assumption: if we restore your weight, everything else will follow. Your thoughts will normalize. Your behaviors will stop. Your brain will heal.

For many autistic women, this framework misses the point entirely. Research shows that for autistic individuals with restrictive eating, weight and body image concerns are often secondary to other factors—sensory sensitivities, need for control, routine adherence, and emotional regulation difficulties (Brede et al., 2020). Yet treatment protocols designed around body image work don't address these core issues.

Consider the standard residential treatment approach: forced weight gain through supervised eating and meal supplements. You're weighed backward (so you can't see the number, but the anxiety about the number remains). Staff monitor bathroom use. Exercise is restricted. Everything focuses on making your body bigger. For a neurotypical person with anorexia nervosa driven by fear of weight gain, this makes sense—you're facing the core fear. But for an autistic woman whose restriction stems from sensory overwhelm, executive function paralysis, or need for predictability? The weight focus doesn't address why you stopped eating in the first place.

Jalila, a 27-year-old autistic woman, spent four months in residential treatment where she gained 25 pounds and was discharged as "weight restored." Within six weeks, she'd lost 20 of those pounds. Her treatment team called this treatment failure and recommended another residential stay. But Jalila's weight loss wasn't about wanting to be thin. At home, without the structured meal plan, she couldn't figure out what to eat. Decision fatigue overwhelmed her. Without staff prompting her at meal times, she forgot to eat. The sensory issues that made eating difficult in the first place—which residential treatment had bypassed through supplements and limited food choices—came flooding back. She'd gained weight, but she hadn't learned to eat as an autistic person in the real world. The weight-focused approach had taught her body to be heavier while ignoring the practical, autism-related barriers to sustained eating.

The weight-focus fallacy extends to how treatment teams interpret behaviors. Autistic traits—need for sameness, sensory sensitivities, rigid routines—get pathologized as eating disorder symptoms requiring elimination. Your need to eat at the same time each day? Eating disorder rigidity. Your difficulty with mixed textures? Avoidance behavior. Your preference for predictable foods? Restriction. Nobody asks: are these autistic traits that actually help you eat consistently? Or are they eating disorder behaviors that need challenging?

Research examining eating disorder treatment outcomes for autistic individuals consistently shows worse outcomes and longer treatment duration compared to non-autistic individuals (Kinnaird et al., 2017). The weight-focused model doesn't account for the reality that autistic bodies and brains have different needs. Recovery for you might mean maintaining adequate nutrition with accommodations for sensory issues, rather than achieving an arbitrary BMI number while ignoring the autism-related factors that affect your eating.

3.2 Group Therapy Exhaustion

Walk into any eating disorder treatment program and you'll find groups. Lots of them. Morning process group, meal support group, body image group, dialectical behavior therapy group, art therapy group, family group. The treatment philosophy: shared experiences create healing. Peer support reduces isolation. Group dynamics facilitate change.

For autistic women, group therapy is often the opposite of therapeutic. The social demands alone are exhausting—reading facial expressions, interpreting tone, knowing when to speak, managing eye contact, following rapid conversational shifts (Babb et al., 2021). Add the content of eating disorder groups—emotional vulnerability, processing feelings, sharing intimate struggles—and the cognitive load becomes overwhelming. You're supposed to focus on recovery, but you're spending all your energy just trying to appear socially competent.

Then there's the sensory environment. Twelve people in a small room. Fluorescent lights. Someone tapping their pen. Another person's strong perfume. Chairs scraping on floors. Multiple conversations happening simultaneously during "pair and share" exercises. For autistic individuals with sensory processing differences, these environments trigger constant low-level stress that makes therapeutic engagement nearly impossible (Tavassoli et al., 2014).

The group therapy format also assumes certain social-emotional skills that many autistic people find challenging. "Notice what comes up for you as Maria shares her experience." "Provide feedback to your partner about the emotions you're observing." "Reflect back what you heard using active listening." These instructions require theory of mind, emotional recognition, and social reciprocity—skills that are specifically impaired in autism (Baron-Cohen, 1997). You're not learning eating disorder recovery skills. You're struggling with social skills deficits while being judged as "not engaging in treatment."

Marcus, a 31-year-old autistic man in a mixed-gender eating disorder program, describes his group therapy experience: "I'd sit there completely overwhelmed, trying to process what people were saying while also monitoring my body language so I didn't seem disengaged. Someone would share something emotional and I'd have no idea how to respond. Should I make sympathetic sounds? Nod? Look concerned? I was so focused on appearing appropriate that I couldn't actually process the content. Then they'd ask me to share and I'd go blank. Not because I had nothing to say, but because I'd used all my energy on the social performance. The therapist wrote in my chart that I was 'resistant to group process' and 'appeared checked out.' I wasn't resistant. I was autistic."

Group meals add another layer of difficulty. You're expected to eat while socializing—two cognitively demanding tasks simultaneously. For many autistic people, eating requires focused attention. You need to monitor hunger cues, manage sensory experiences of food, pace yourself appropriately. Adding social demands makes eating exponentially harder. Research shows that autistic individuals eat significantly less in social contexts compared to eating alone (Lucarelli et al., 2017). Yet eating disorder programs structure meals as social events, then interpret your reduced intake as eating disorder behavior rather than autism-related social eating difficulty.

3.3 CBT's Pattern Problem

Cognitive Behavioral Therapy (CBT) is the gold standard treatment for eating disorders. The model makes logical sense: identify distorted thoughts, challenge them with evidence, replace them with balanced thoughts, and behaviors change. Works beautifully for many people. For autistic individuals, it often doesn't.

Standard CBT for eating disorders targets specific cognitive distortions. "I feel fat" is challenged as a feeling, not a fact. "Eating this will make me gain five pounds" is challenged as catastrophizing. "I can only eat safe foods" is challenged as black-and-white thinking. The therapy assumes these thoughts are irrational distortions requiring correction.

But autistic thinking doesn't always fit the distortion model. When an autistic woman says "I can only eat these specific foods," that might not be a cognitive distortion—it might be an accurate assessment of her sensory system's limitations (Kinnaird et al., 2019). When she insists on eating at the same time each day, that's not necessarily pathological rigidity—it might be adaptive routine that reduces anxiety and supports consistent eating. Traditional CBT pathologizes autism traits as eating disorder symptoms.

The cognitive challenging process itself poses problems for autistic thinking styles. CBT relies on recognizing thoughts as "just thoughts"—mental events you can observe and evaluate. Many autistic people think in concrete, literal patterns. A thought isn't a mental event to be evaluated; it's a fact about reality. The metacognitive skills CBT requires—thinking about thinking—don't come naturally to concrete, pattern-based processors (Russell, 1997).

Sofia, a 24-year-old autistic graduate student, spent eight months in CBT for her eating disorder. Each session, her therapist had her identify distorted thoughts about food and challenge them. "Carbs are dangerous" became "carbs are a normal part of a balanced diet—distorted thinking." But Sofia wasn't catastrophizing about carbs. She'd read research linking processed carbohydrates to inflammation and had created rules based on that information. Her thoughts followed logical patterns from premises she accepted. The therapist kept treating her pattern-based reasoning as distortion requiring correction. Sofia would agree intellectually that carbs weren't dangerous, then go home and follow her rules because the logical chain that created them still made sense to her. After months of CBT, her therapist concluded she was "treatment resistant." Actually, she was autistic, and the treatment model didn't match how her brain processed information.

This isn't to say cognitive approaches can't help autistic people. They can. But they need adaptation. Instead of challenging "distorted" thoughts, therapy needs to help autistic individuals distinguish between thoughts that serve their wellbeing and thoughts that serve the eating disorder. Some rigid rules help you eat consistently. Others restrict you unnecessarily. The work isn't eliminating all food rules—it's developing discernment about which rules support health and which don't.

3.4 Exposure Therapy Overload

Exposure therapy is a core component of eating disorder treatment. You're systematically exposed to fear foods, challenging situations, and anxiety-provoking experiences. The theory: avoidance maintains anxiety. Facing fears reduces anxiety through habituation. Eat the pizza repeatedly, and eventually pizza stops feeling terrifying.

For many autistic individuals, exposure therapy as practiced in eating disorder settings creates more trauma than healing. Standard exposure protocols push you to tolerate distress until anxiety decreases. But if your distress comes from genuine sensory overload rather than irrational fear, habituation doesn't happen. You're not getting used to the food. You're repeatedly triggering your nervous system's threat response without relief.

Consider a standard exposure exercise: eating a previously avoided food in a challenging environment. Maybe pizza in a crowded restaurant. For a neurotypical person with anorexia whose fear is primarily about calories and weight gain, this exposure makes therapeutic sense. Facing the fear demonstrates that eating pizza doesn't result in catastrophic weight gain. But for an autistic person whose pizza avoidance stems from sensory issues with melted cheese, loud restaurant environments, and unpredictable social demands, this exposure is just traumatic. You're not learning that pizza is safe. You're learning that treatment is torturous.

The pace of exposure in eating disorder programs often ignores autistic processing needs. Standard protocols move quickly—you might be expected to try multiple fear foods per week. But autistic nervous systems often need more time to process new experiences. What looks like "avoidance" or "resistance" might be your brain requiring additional processing time before integrating a new food (Kinnaird et al., 2019).

Treatment teams also struggle to distinguish between eating disorder fear and autism-related distress. Both can look like food refusal. Both can trigger anxiety. But the intervention differs significantly. Eating disorder fear benefits from exposure and habituation. Autism-related sensory distress requires accommodations and gradual desensitization using different techniques. Pushing exposure when accommodation is needed causes harm.

Amina, a 29-year-old autistic woman, was required to eat yogurt as part of her exposure protocol. She'd avoided yogurt her entire life due to texture issues—the slimy, slippery consistency triggered immediate gag reflexes. Her treatment team interpreted this as eating disorder avoidance and insisted she practice exposures. Each attempt ended with Amina gagging, sometimes vomiting, feeling overwhelmed and ashamed. The team's response: "You need to push through the discomfort. Anxiety always decreases with exposure." Except her distress wasn't anxiety. It was a genuine sensory response. After weeks of failed exposures, Amina felt more traumatized and less trusting of treatment. Eventually, a therapist with autism training recognized the sensory component and stopped the yogurt exposures. Instead, they worked on expanding other food options that didn't trigger sensory distress. Amina made more progress in two months than she had in the previous six months of forced exposures.

Hospital and residential programs add environmental sensory challenges that compound exposure difficulties. Bright lights, constant noise, lack of private space, unpredictable schedules, strong cleaning product smells—all of these create baseline sensory stress that makes food exposure even harder (Tavassoli et al., 2014). You're supposed to face food fears while your nervous system is already maxed out from environmental overload.

3.5 Intuitive Eating Impossibility

"Listen to your body. Eat when you're hungry. Stop when you're full. Honor your cravings." Intuitive eating has become a cornerstone of eating disorder recovery, particularly for those moving beyond rigid meal plans. The philosophy makes sense: reconnect with your body's natural signals, trust your internal wisdom, let go of external rules.

For autistic individuals with interoception difficulties, intuitive eating is functionally impossible—at least initially. As we discussed in section 2.2, interoception—the ability to sense internal body signals—is impaired in approximately 70% of autistic adults (DuBois et al., 2016). When you can't reliably detect hunger or fullness, "listening to your body" is meaningless advice. It's like telling someone who's colorblind to paint by observing subtle color variations.

Standard eating disorder recovery programs eventually transition patients from structured meal plans to intuitive eating. The assumption: structure is training wheels. Real recovery means eating freely based on body cues. But for autistic people, structure isn't training wheels—it's the accommodation that makes eating possible. Removing structure without alternative supports sets up failure.

The intuitive eating framework also assumes that removing external rules allows natural, balanced eating to emerge. For autistic brains wired for pattern-based thinking and rule-following, removing all rules often creates paralysis rather than freedom. Without guidelines, decision-making becomes overwhelming. Executive function challenges make "figure it out as you go" approaches extremely difficult (Demetriou et al., 2018).

Think about what intuitive eating requires moment-to-moment. Notice subtle hunger signals. Distinguish hunger from other uncomfortable sensations. Decide what your body needs. Choose foods based on that need. Notice emerging fullness. Stop eating at comfortable fullness. Each step requires interoceptive accuracy and executive function. For many autistic people, this entire sequence is impaired.

Diego, a 26-year-old autistic man, describes his experience with intuitive eating: "My dietitian kept saying 'get curious about what your body wants.' But my body doesn't tell me what it wants. Sometimes I'm lightheaded and irritable and don't realize I haven't eaten in eight hours. Other times I eat because it's a scheduled meal time, not because I feel hungry. When I tried intuitive eating, I'd stand in front of the refrigerator for 20 minutes unable to decide what to eat. Or I'd eat way too much because I couldn't detect fullness until I felt physically sick. It wasn't freeing. It was chaos. Going back to a structured meal plan actually helped me eat more consistently."

This doesn't mean autistic people can't develop better interoception or more flexible eating patterns. They can. But the path isn't through immediately abandoning structure for intuition. It's through gradually building interoceptive awareness while maintaining enough structure to ensure adequate nutrition. It's developing personalized guidelines that work with autistic processing styles rather than against them.

3.6 Hospital Sensory Nightmares

Residential eating disorder programs and hospital settings are designed for safety and structure. What they're not designed for is sensory sensitivity. For autistic individuals, these environments can be so sensorially overwhelming that recovery becomes nearly impossible.

Start with the visual environment. Fluorescent lights—the kind that flicker at frequencies most people don't consciously notice but that autistic nervous systems process as constant strobing (Tavassoli et al., 2014). White walls reflecting harsh light. Limited access to natural light. Visual clutter in common spaces. For someone with visual sensory sensitivities, these environments create constant low-level stress.

Then there's sound. Residential programs are loud. Multiple people in shared spaces. TV in common rooms. Staff conversations. Doors closing. Announcements over intercoms. Meal times with utensils clanking, multiple conversations, chairs moving. For autistic individuals with auditory sensitivities, this constant noise is torture. You can't escape it. Quiet spaces are limited or non-existent. Noise-canceling headphones might be forbidden due to safety concerns. You're trapped in auditory overload.

Smell poses another challenge. Institutional cleaning products. Other residents' perfumes or hygiene products. Food smells from the kitchen. Hand sanitizer. For those with olfactory sensitivities, these smells can trigger nausea, headaches, or overwhelming discomfort. You're supposed to eat and focus on recovery while your olfactory system is in distress.

The lack of control over your environment compounds these challenges. You can't adjust the lights. You can't control the temperature (often too cold or too warm). You can't choose when to be around people versus alone. Your schedule is dictated—wake times, meal times, group times, bed times. For autistic individuals who rely on environmental control to manage sensory processing, this loss of agency is destabilizing (Kinnaird et al., 2017).

Chen, a 33-year-old autistic software engineer, spent six weeks in residential treatment. She describes it as "sensory torture masquerading as healing." The fluorescent lights gave her migraines. The constant noise made sleep nearly impossible. The smell of industrial cleaning products made her nauseous. She couldn't eat in the dining room because the sensory overload was too extreme—but refusing to eat in the dining room was documented as "eating disorder behavior" and "lack of treatment engagement." She asked for accommodations—dimmer lights in her room, a quieter space to eat, permission to use noise-canceling headphones. Each request was denied or required extensive justification. She left treatment early, labeled treatment-resistant, when actually she was an autistic person in an environment incompatible with her neurology.

The irony: programs designed to help you eat create environments where sensory overload makes eating significantly harder. You're already struggling with food. Adding constant sensory distress ensures failure for many autistic individuals.

3.7 The Accommodation Revolution

So what do autistic individuals with eating disorders actually need? Not compliance with standard protocols. Accommodation and adaptation.

Sensory accommodations: Dimmed lights, quiet eating spaces, reduced olfactory triggers, temperature control, access to sensory tools (headphones, fidgets, weighted blankets), and permission to eat alone when group settings are overwhelming. These aren't special privileges—they're necessary supports that allow autistic nervous systems to function well enough to engage in recovery (Tchanturia et al., 2020).

Modified group therapy: Smaller groups, clear agendas provided in advance, explicit social expectations, frequent breaks, and understanding that reduced eye contact or limited verbal participation don't equal lack of engagement. Better yet, individual therapy as the primary modality with optional groups rather than mandatory daily group attendance.

Adapted cognitive approaches: Working with pattern-based thinking rather than against it. Helping distinguish helpful rules from harmful ones instead of eliminating all food rules. Using concrete, logical frameworks instead of abstract emotional processing. Building on autistic thinking strengths rather than pathologizing them.

Structured eating plans: Maintaining meal structure throughout recovery, not as a temporary measure but as a permanent accommodation for interoception difficulties. Creating personalized guidelines that reduce decision fatigue while supporting nutritional adequacy.

Sensory-informed exposure: Gradual, autistic-paced exposure that distinguishes sensory distress from eating disorder fear. Accommodating genuine sensory needs while still expanding food variety through adapted techniques. Never forcing exposure that creates trauma.

Routine flexibility training: Teaching graduated flexibility within structure rather than eliminating structure entirely. The goal isn't "normal" spontaneous eating—it's flexible enough to eat in various circumstances while maintaining enough routine to support consistent eating.

Executive function support: Explicit meal planning strategies, simplified food preparation, external reminders and prompts, and reducing the cognitive demands of eating so limited executive function resources go toward actually eating rather than planning what to eat.

Research on the PEACE Pathway—an eating disorder treatment program specifically adapted for autistic individuals—demonstrates that these accommodations work (Tchanturia et al., 2020). Autistic patients receiving adapted treatment showed comparable or better outcomes than non-autistic patients receiving standard treatment. The difference wasn't that autistic people suddenly became easier to treat. The difference was that treatment finally addressed their actual needs.

3.8 What You Deserve

You deserved treatment that saw your autism from day one. You deserved clinicians who understood that your need for routine wasn't eating disorder rigidity. You deserved sensory accommodations that allowed your nervous system to regulate well enough to eat. You deserved cognitive approaches that worked with your thinking style. You deserved to not be labeled treatment-resistant when the treatment was autism-inappropriate.

If past treatment failed you, it likely wasn't your fault. Standard eating disorder treatment wasn't designed for autistic brains. The failure was in the treatment model, not in you.

Recovery is possible for autistic individuals with eating disorders. But it requires treatment that accommodates autism while addressing the eating disorder. It requires clinicians who understand the intersection of these conditions. It requires adaptations, not just compliance.

The following chapters provide specific strategies for building your own autism-accommodated recovery. You'll learn to work with your sensory system, develop appropriate structure that supports rather than restricts eating, and create flexibility within your autistic neurology. Recovery doesn't mean becoming neurotypical. It means eating consistently and adequately as the autistic person you are.

Chapter 4.0: Building Your Sensory Safe World

Your relationship with food starts with your sensory system. Before thoughts about calories enter your mind, before anxiety kicks in, your nervous system processes the sensory reality of eating—how food looks, smells, feels in your mouth, sounds when you chew it, tastes on your tongue. For autistic individuals, this sensory processing often works differently. Some sensations feel more intense. Others barely register. Certain textures trigger immediate disgust while others feel comforting.

This chapter helps you understand your unique sensory profile and build a food world that works with your neurology instead of fighting against it. You'll learn to expand your food options gradually without triggering the restriction patterns that eating disorders thrive on. The goal isn't forcing yourself to eat everything—it's creating enough variety for nutritional adequacy while respecting genuine sensory limitations.

4.1 Your Personal Sensory Audit

Before changing anything, you need to understand your current sensory relationship with food. This isn't about judgment or shame. It's about gathering accurate information. Think of it like running diagnostics on your computer—you're identifying how your system actually works, not how it's supposed to work.

Start by listing the foods you currently eat comfortably. Not foods you force down. Not foods you eat because they're "safe" from an eating disorder perspective. Foods that feel genuinely okay in your sensory system. For some people, this list might include 30 foods. For others, five. Both are valid starting points.

For each food on your list, identify what makes it sensorially acceptable. Consider:

Texture: Is it smooth? Crunchy? Soft? Firm? Does it maintain consistent texture throughout, or does it change as you chew? Mixed texture foods—like soup with chunks, salad with different components, sandwiches with multiple layers—often pose more challenges for autistic sensory systems than uniform texture foods (Cermak et al., 2010).

Temperature: Do you prefer foods cold, room temperature, hot? Some autistic individuals have strong temperature preferences that others might not notice. Maybe you can eat chicken cold but not hot. Maybe raw vegetables work but cooked ones don't. These aren't random preferences—they're sensory patterns.

Visual appearance: Color matters more than most people realize. Research shows that autistic children often avoid foods based on color patterns (Nadon et al., 2011). Maybe you only eat beige/brown foods. Maybe bright colors feel overwhelming. Maybe irregular shapes bother you but uniform shapes feel acceptable.

Smell: What does each safe food smell like? Strong smells versus mild? Certain smell categories (meaty, dairy, sweet, starchy) more acceptable than others? Olfactory sensitivities in autism can be intense—some smells that others find pleasant or neutral might trigger nausea or headaches for you (Bennetto et al., 2007).

Sound: Yes, sound matters. The crunch of chips, the squish of bananas, the crackle of cereal in milk. Some autistic people strongly prefer crunchy foods partly because of the auditory feedback. Others avoid crunchy foods for the same reason—the sound overwhelms them.

Flavor complexity: Simple, single flavors versus complex flavor combinations? Mild versus strong? Certain autistic individuals prefer foods with clear, predictable flavors rather than complex dishes where multiple flavors compete (Nadon et al., 2011).

Now do the same exercise for foods you currently avoid. What specific sensory properties make them intolerable? Be detailed. "I don't like mushrooms" isn't specific enough. "I don't like mushrooms because they're slimy, rubbery, and the texture changes unpredictably when you chew them" gives you actionable information.

This audit reveals your sensory patterns. Maybe you're okay with any temperature but struggle with mixed textures. Maybe visual appearance doesn't bother you but smell is a deal-breaker. Maybe you handle most things fine except slimy or stringy textures. These patterns guide how you expand your food world.

4.2 Expanding Foods Without Restriction Patterns

Here's the tricky part: eating disorders love limited food variety. Restriction thrives when you eat the same few foods repeatedly. But forcing yourself to eat sensorially distressing foods feeds into eating disorder mentality too—the "just push through it" thinking that ignores your body's genuine needs.

The solution isn't choosing between eating disorder restriction and sensory torture. It's strategic expansion that respects sensory boundaries while gradually increasing variety.

Identify "bridge foods": These are foods similar enough to your safe foods that your sensory system might tolerate them, but different enough to add variety. If you eat chicken nuggets comfortably, a bridge food might be baked chicken strips—similar texture, shape, and flavor but slightly different preparation. If you eat white rice, maybe jasmine rice or brown rice becomes a bridge option. The sensory jump is small enough that habituation is possible (Fraker et al., 2007).

Use the "one change rule": When trying to expand, change only one sensory variable at a time. If you eat cold, plain pasta with butter, maybe try cold, plain pasta with olive oil (same temperature, same plainness, different fat). Once that's comfortable, try warm pasta with olive oil (same fat, same plainness, different temperature). Changing multiple variables simultaneously overwhelms sensory processing.

Distinguish eating disorder restriction from sensory accommodation: This requires brutal honesty. Are you avoiding a food because it genuinely triggers sensory distress? Or because your eating disorder has labeled it dangerous? Sometimes both are true—the eating disorder co-opts genuine sensory sensitivities to justify restriction. Working with a therapist who understands both autism and eating disorders helps distinguish these patterns.

Elena, a 30-year-old autistic woman recovering from anorexia, realized her food avoidance had two distinct sources. She genuinely couldn't tolerate yogurt—the slimy texture triggered immediate gagging regardless of recovery motivation. That was sensory. But she also avoided bread, claiming texture issues, when really she feared carbohydrates. When she tried bread in a safe context with support, she found the texture actually felt fine. Her brain had created a false sensory rationale to mask eating disorder fear. Once she distinguished genuine sensory issues from eating disorder manipulation of sensory language, she could address each appropriately. Yogurt stayed off her list as a legitimate sensory accommodation. Bread gradually returned through exposure.

Track your progress without obsessing: Keep a simple log of new foods you try. This prevents memory distortion where you think you've tried nothing new when you've actually tried five things. But don't turn this into rigid rules about "must try X new foods per week." Recovery pacing varies. Some weeks you'll expand. Other weeks you'll maintain. Both are acceptable.

4.3 Texture Temperature and Color Work

Let's get specific about the sensory properties that create the most challenges for autistic eaters: texture, temperature, and color.

Texture hierarchy: Most people find certain texture categories more challenging than others. Common difficult textures for autistic individuals include slimy (okra, oysters, overcooked eggs), rubbery (some meats, mushrooms), stringy (melted cheese, celery), mixed consistency (yogurt with fruit chunks), and foods that change texture dramatically when chewed (tomatoes) (Nadon et al., 2011). Identifying which texture categories feel most distressing helps you understand your expansion path.

If slimy is your worst category, you don't need to ever make peace with oysters. That's okay. You can get adequate nutrition without oysters. But maybe you can expand within crunchy textures if those feel more tolerable. Focus expansion efforts on sensory categories that feel less distressing.

Some texture challenges have workarounds. If you struggle with mixed textures, eat components separately. If ground meat's texture bothers you, try firmer cuts. If vegetables' texture feels wrong when cooked, try them raw. Your eating doesn't need to look like everyone else's eating.

Temperature strategies: Temperature sensitivity affects more autistic eaters than most clinicians realize. Some people can only eat foods cold. Others need everything hot. Many can't tolerate foods that should be hot served cold, or vice versa (Nadon et al., 2011).

If temperature matters to you, honor it. Eat ice cream melted if that's what works. Eat pizza cold if hot pizza's temperature overwhelms you. Eat cold cuts heated if that's your preference. Society's rules about "proper" food temperatures are arbitrary. Your nervous system's needs are not.

Temperature also offers an expansion avenue. If you eat something cold comfortably, try it room temperature. Then warm. Then hot. Or reverse the progression. Small temperature shifts are easier than big ones.

Color considerations: This sounds superficial until you experience it. Some autistic individuals can only eat beige/brown foods—chicken, bread, crackers, pasta, potatoes. The visual input of brightly colored foods creates discomfort that overrides any rational knowledge that color doesn't affect nutrition (Nadon et al., 2011).

If color affects you, work with it, not against it. Start with foods close to colors you already accept. If beige is comfortable, maybe tan or light yellow becomes acceptable before you move to orange or green. Some people never expand color tolerance much, and that's okay. You can meet nutritional needs with limited color variety.

Mixing colors can also help. If plain green broccoli feels overwhelming, maybe broccoli mixed into beige pasta becomes tolerable because the color impact is reduced. Or covering challenging-colored foods with acceptable-colored sauces might work. These aren't tricks or avoidance—they're accommodations that make eating possible.

4.4 The Gentle Exposure Method

Traditional exposure therapy for eating disorders pushes rapid confrontation with fear foods. For autistic sensory sensitivities, this approach often traumatizes rather than desensitizes. You need a gentler method that respects how autistic nervous systems process new sensory information.

The progression approach: Instead of jumping straight to eating a challenging food, create graduated steps:

1. **Visual exposure**: Have the food present in the room without eating it. Look at it. Notice your reaction.
2. **Olfactory exposure**: Smell the food. Notice how your body responds. This step is crucial—smell often triggers rejection before taste.
3. **Touch exposure**: Touch the food with your hands. How does it feel?
4. **Taste exposure**: Lick the food or take a tiny taste without swallowing. What information does your sensory system give you?

5. **Small bite**: Chew and swallow a small piece. Notice the full sensory experience.
6. **Regular portion**: Work up to eating a normal serving.

Don't rush through these steps. Each might take days or weeks. That's fine. You're teaching your nervous system that this food is safe, not forcing compliance through willpower.

Pairing with safe foods: Eating a challenging food alongside a safe, comforting food reduces anxiety. If you're trying to introduce strawberries (difficult due to texture and seeds), eat them alongside your safest food—maybe crackers. The familiar sensory experience of the safe food provides nervous system regulation while you process the new food.

Time and context matter: Try new foods when you're otherwise regulated—not when you're already overwhelmed, rushed, or stressed. Late afternoon after a restful day works better than early morning when you're already managing the sensory assault of getting ready for work. Choose low-pressure contexts without social demands or time constraints.

Respect genuine "no": Sometimes after multiple exposures, your body still says no to a food. That's information, not failure. Some textures might never become tolerable. Sensory processing differences are neurological, not just psychological. Habituation works for many textures, but not all. When habituation isn't happening despite gentle, repeated exposure, that food might genuinely be outside your sensory tolerance range. That's okay. Move on to other expansion options.

Marcus, a 28-year-old autistic man, spent three months trying to introduce tomatoes using gentle exposure. He could look at them fine. Touching them felt okay. But the moment tomato taste entered his mouth, he experienced immediate nausea and strong urge to spit it out. After multiple attempts using every strategy—pairing with safe foods, trying different tomato preparations, adjusting context—his sensory system still rejected tomatoes. His dietitian finally said,

"You don't have to eat tomatoes. We can meet your nutritional needs other ways." That permission to stop trying felt like relief, not failure. Marcus's energy went toward successfully introducing bell peppers instead, which his sensory system accepted more readily.

4.5 Routines That Support Recovery

Autistic brains thrive on routine. Eating disorder brains thrive on rigid rules. How do you create eating routines that support recovery without feeding restriction?

Structured flexibility: This might sound contradictory, but it's the sweet spot. You need enough structure to reduce decision fatigue and support consistent eating, but enough flexibility to eat in imperfect circumstances. Structure looks like eating at roughly the same times each day—not exactly 8:00, 12:00, and 6:00, but within a reasonable window. Flexibility looks like being able to eat your morning meal between 7:00 and 9:00 depending on your schedule.

Meal rotation systems: Instead of eating the exact same thing every day (eating disorder rigidity), create a rotation of 5-7 acceptable breakfast options, 5-7 lunch options, and 5-7 dinner options. You're choosing from a defined set, which reduces decision paralysis, but you're not locked into identical meals daily, which prevents the monotony that often triggers bingeing or restriction patterns (Fraker et al., 2007).

Environmental consistency: Where you eat matters for autistic nervous systems. Eating in the same location—your kitchen table, a specific chair, a particular room—creates environmental predictability that supports eating. This is different from eating disorder rituals that serve restriction. You're providing your nervous system with familiar cues that signal "this is eating time."

Sensory-friendly eating environment: Make your eating space as sensorially comfortable as possible. Reduce visual clutter. Minimize background noise or use pleasant background sound if silence feels wrong. Control lighting—maybe softer lighting feels better than harsh overhead lights. Remove strong smells. These environmental supports make the sensory demands of eating itself more manageable.

Time boundaries without obsession: Meals need some time structure—you can't graze all day because hunger cues are unreliable. But timing doesn't need to be rigid. "Breakfast happens within an hour of waking" is structure. "Breakfast must be at 8:00 AM or I've failed" is eating disorder rigidity. Learn to tell the difference.

4.6 Meal Planning That Works

Executive function challenges make meal planning genuinely difficult for many autistic people, as we discussed in section 2.3. When you add eating disorder recovery on top of executive function difficulties, meal planning can feel impossible. Here are strategies that actually work.

Template-based planning: Instead of deciding from scratch what to eat, use meal templates. Breakfast template: protein + starch + fat. Lunch template: protein + vegetable + starch + fat. Dinner template: same as lunch. Within each template, rotate options. This eliminates most decision-making while ensuring nutritional variety (Nadon et al., 2011).

Batch preparation: Executive function struggles often show up most intensely around food preparation, not eating itself. Making decisions about what to cook, following recipes with multiple steps, managing timing—all of these overwhelm executive function. Batch preparation helps. Cook multiple servings at once when executive function is relatively intact. Refrigerate or freeze portions. Reheat when you're too overwhelmed to cook from scratch.

Pre-portioned options: Having to figure out appropriate portions requires working memory and decision-making when you're already hungry and potentially dysregulated. Pre-portioned foods—individual yogurts, pre-cut vegetables, single-serve containers—

eliminate portion decisions. Yes, they're more expensive. They're also an accommodation that makes eating possible.

Visual meal planning tools: Many autistic people think visually better than verbally. Instead of a written meal plan, use pictures. Take photos of meals you eat comfortably. Create a visual meal plan by arranging these photos into daily combinations. Some people use Pinterest boards or photo apps. Visual planning reduces the verbal-processing demands that written meal plans require.

External reminders: You will forget to eat. That's not moral failure. That's poor interoception plus executive function challenges. Set phone alarms for meal and snack times. Use reminder apps. Ask trusted people to check in. These external scaffolds replace unreliable internal signals.

Priya, a 33-year-old autistic attorney, struggled with meal planning throughout her eating disorder. Trying to follow a written meal plan felt overwhelming—she'd stare at the list unable to translate "3 oz protein, 1 cup vegetable, 1 cup grain" into actual food. She worked with her dietitian to create a visual meal plan. They photographed 20 different meals Priya could comfortably eat. Using these photos, Priya arranged her weekly meals visually on her phone. Instead of reading and interpreting a written plan, she looked at the photo and replicated that meal. This simple accommodation made consistent eating possible for the first time in years.

4.7 Accommodating Sensory Needs Carefully

Here's where things get nuanced. You need sensory accommodations to eat consistently. But eating disorders can disguise themselves as sensory needs. How do you accommodate genuine sensory challenges without enabling restriction?

Test your accommodations: A legitimate sensory accommodation allows you to eat more consistently with better nutrition. An eating disorder restriction disguised as sensory need results in eating less or with reduced variety. If your "accommodation" means you're eating less than before, it's probably not a real accommodation.

Compare past and present: Were these sensory issues present before your eating disorder? Did you avoid these textures in childhood? If sensory avoidance is genuinely autism-related, it typically predates the eating disorder. If suddenly all warm foods feel intolerable right after you developed an eating disorder, that's worth examining more critically.

Check the fear content: Sensory distress feels physically uncomfortable—gag reflex, nausea, sensory overwhelm. Eating disorder fear feels psychologically uncomfortable—anxiety, guilt, fear of consequences. They're different nervous system responses. Get honest about which you're experiencing. If you think a food will "feel wrong" but actually you're afraid of what eating it means for your body or weight, that's eating disorder fear wearing a sensory mask.

Use the "just structure" test: If someone else structured your eating completely—told you exactly what to eat, when to eat, handled all preparation, and you just had to eat the food—could you do it? If the answer is "yes, if it meets my sensory needs" but you can't manage it when you're responsible for planning and preparation, you're dealing primarily with executive function challenges, not sensory issues. That distinction matters for intervention.

Work with knowledgeable professionals: Distinguishing genuine sensory accommodation from eating disorder manipulation is difficult alone. A therapist or dietitian who understands both autism and eating disorders can help you evaluate whether specific accommodations support recovery or enable restriction. This isn't about judgment—it's about accurate assessment.

4.8 Creating Your Food World

Your sensory-safe food world doesn't need to include every food. It needs to include enough variety for nutritional adequacy and enough flexibility for eating in different contexts. What "enough" means varies individually.

Some autistic people recover eating 40 different foods. Others recover eating 15. Both can be nutritionally adequate if those foods cover necessary macronutrients and micronutrients. Your goal isn't matching someone else's variety. It's finding your sustainable variety—foods your sensory system tolerates consistently enough to support health.

Think about contexts where you need to eat: at home, at work, at friends' or family's homes, at restaurants, while traveling. You need at least a few options that work in each context. This might mean building a "restaurant safe foods" list of items available at most restaurants that meet your sensory needs. Or packing your own food when visiting others. Or finding portable safe foods for travel.

Recovery means having enough food options to fuel your life adequately. That's the standard. Not gourmet variety. Not adventurous eating. Not Instagram-worthy meals. Adequate nutrition that works with your autistic sensory processing.

Building your sensory-safe food world is ongoing work. Your tolerance might expand over time. Or it might not. Both outcomes are acceptable. The goal is eating consistently as the autistic person you are, sensory sensitivities and all.

4.9 Essential Points to Remember

Sensory processing differences aren't personality flaws requiring correction—they're neurological realities requiring accommodation. Your recovery involves working with your sensory system, not forcing it into submission. By understanding your specific sensory patterns, creating gentle exposure pathways, establishing supportive routines, and accommodating genuine sensory needs while challenging eating disorder restriction, you build a food world that sustains you.

The strategies in this chapter help you expand your food options without traumatizing your nervous system or enabling eating disorder restriction. Remember: adequate nutrition with sensory accommodations is recovery. You don't need to eat everything. You need to eat enough of the right things consistently. That's entirely possible within your autistic sensory processing.

Chapter 5.0: Rewiring Rigid Thinking

Your brain loves patterns. Rules. Predictability. This is autism doing what autism does—creating structure to make sense of an unpredictable world. It's one of your cognitive strengths. Pattern recognition, systematic thinking, attention to detail—these skills serve you well in many areas of life. But when eating disorders hijack your pattern-based thinking, those same cognitive strengths become vulnerabilities. Rules that started as helpful structure become restrictive prisons. Patterns that reduce anxiety become rigid compulsions. Your brain's natural preference for sameness amplifies eating disorder behaviors in ways that make traditional recovery approaches ineffective.

This chapter teaches you to work with autistic thinking patterns while breaking free from eating disorder rigidity. You'll learn to distinguish structure that supports you from rules that restrict you. You'll develop enough cognitive flexibility to eat in imperfect circumstances without losing the routines your autistic brain needs. This is the hardest balance in autism-eating disorder recovery, but it's also the most critical.

5.1 Pattern Thinking in Eating Disorders

Autistic cognition tends toward systemizing—seeking patterns, creating rules, following logical structures (Baron-Cohen, 2009). This thinking style excels at mathematics, programming, categorization, and detailed analysis. It struggles with ambiguity, unpredictability, and situations without clear rules.

When diet culture enters your life with its endless proclamations—"carbs are bad," "eat six small meals," "no eating after 7 PM," "always eat breakfast"—your pattern-seeking brain latches onto these rules with intensity. They offer clear structure in the inherently ambiguous domain of "what should I eat?" Your brain experiences relief finding rules where before there was only confusion and social complexity.

Research on cognitive flexibility in autism shows that autistic individuals demonstrate more difficulty shifting between tasks, adapting to rule changes, and generating alternative solutions compared to neurotypical individuals (Dajani & Uddin, 2015). This cognitive profile means that once your brain accepts a food rule as true, questioning or abandoning that rule feels nearly impossible. The rule becomes part of your mental operating system.

Eating disorders exploit this. They present as helpful systems: "Follow these rules and you'll be safe." "This structure gives you control." Your autistic brain, already wired for rule-based thinking, finds this message compelling. What starts as one or two rules proliferates. No eating after 6 PM becomes no eating after 5 PM becomes only eating within a four-hour window. No dessert on weekdays becomes no dessert ever becomes no foods with added sugar. The eating disorder exploits your cognitive style's greatest strength—pattern recognition and rule adherence—against you.

Here's what makes this particularly insidious: some of your food rules actually help you. Eating at consistent times supports your need for routine and compensates for poor interoception. Having structured meal plans reduces executive function demands. Your brain can't easily distinguish between helpful rules and harmful rules because both provide the psychological comfort of structure. As we discussed in section 3.3, traditional CBT approaches often pathologize all food rules as eating disorder symptoms without recognizing that autistic brains genuinely benefit from some structure (Russell, 1997).

Aisha, a 25-year-old autistic woman, developed anorexia in college. She created an elaborate rule system around eating: certain foods only on certain days, specific meal timing, precise portion measurements, designated eating locations. When treatment pushed her to "be flexible" and "break your rules," she experienced overwhelming anxiety and actually ate less. Her therapist concluded she was treatment-resistant. A new therapist with autism training took a different approach: they categorized Aisha's rules into three groups: rules that supported consistent eating (like eating at scheduled times), rules that restricted unnecessarily (like never eating dessert), and rules that served neither purpose (like only eating in specific locations). They kept the first category, gradually challenged the second, and eventually eliminated the third. This nuanced approach worked because it recognized that Aisha needed some structure—just not eating disorder structure.

5.2 The All or Nothing Problem

All-or-nothing thinking—also called black-and-white thinking or dichotomous thinking—is a cognitive pattern where situations, behaviors, or outcomes are categorized as entirely good or entirely bad with no middle ground (Antony et al., 2007). This thinking style is more common in both autism and eating disorders than in the general population. When these conditions co-occur, all-or-nothing thinking intensifies dramatically.

Food gets sorted into rigid categories: safe and unsafe, good and bad, allowed and forbidden. You're either "being good" (following all rules perfectly) or "failing" (breaking any rule). Meals are either complete successes or total disasters. Recovery means either achieving perfect intuitive eating or remaining sick—no partial progress exists in your mental framework.

This thinking pattern makes recovery brutally difficult. You eat one bite beyond your plan and conclude the entire day is ruined. You try a fear food, experience anxiety, and decide you can never eat it again. You break one rule and think you've destroyed all progress. There's no gradual improvement, no learning curve, no "mostly successful with room for growth." Everything is all or nothing.

The autism component amplifies this. Autistic thinking often lacks the natural gray-zone processing that neurotypical brains employ automatically (Brosnan et al., 2016). You see categories, not spectrums. Boundaries, not gradients. When someone says "eat when you're hungry," your brain wants a rule: exactly how hungry? What are the criteria? Instead of an approximate internal sense, you want clear parameters. When parameters don't exist, anxiety increases. So you create rigid rules to eliminate ambiguity.

Here's how to escape the all-or-nothing trap:

Create middle categories: Instead of just "safe" and "unsafe" foods, develop categories like "always comfortable," "usually okay," "sometimes manageable," "need support to eat," and "genuinely intolerable." This creates gradients instead of dichotomies.

Measure success on a scale: Rate each meal 0-10 for how well it went rather than labeling it success or failure. A meal where you ate adequately despite anxiety? Maybe a seven. A meal where you ate less than planned but didn't restrict entirely? Maybe a five. Nothing is complete success or complete failure.

Use percentage thinking: Instead of "I have to follow my meal plan perfectly," think "I'm aiming for 80-90% adherence most weeks." Perfect adherence isn't the goal. Adequate consistency is.

Build in planned flexibility: Schedule specific times when you deliberately vary your routine slightly. "Wednesday dinner can happen between 5:30 and 7:00" creates intentional gray area. You're practicing flexibility within structure.

Challenge dichotomous language: Notice when you use all-or-nothing words—always, never, completely, totally, perfect, ruined. Mentally replace them with gradient words—usually, rarely, mostly, somewhat, partially, recovering. Language shapes thinking. Changing your words gradually changes your thinking patterns (Antony et al., 2007).

5.3 Building Cognitive Flexibility Carefully

Cognitive flexibility—the ability to adapt thinking and behavior to changing circumstances—is specifically challenging for autistic brains (Dajani & Uddin, 2015). But it's not impossible to develop. It requires different strategies than typical cognitive flexibility training.

Standard cognitive flexibility work involves throwing people into unpredictable situations and expecting adaptation. For autistic individuals, this approach usually triggers overwhelm and shutdown, not flexibility. You need graduated flexibility training that respects your need for predictability while slowly expanding your tolerance for variation.

Predictable unpredictability: This sounds contradictory, but it works. Create scheduled times when you practice small variations. "Every Saturday, I eat breakfast at a different time than usual" or "Once a week, I eat one meal outside my standard rotation." You're still following a rule (practice variation on Saturdays), but the rule involves flexibility. Your brain gets predictability (knowing when flexibility is required) and flexibility practice (actually varying your behavior).

Variation within structure: Keep the structure but vary the details. If your breakfast template is protein + starch + fat, keep that structure but rotate which specific proteins, starches, and fats you choose. Structure provides the framework your autistic brain needs. Variation within that structure builds flexibility without triggering total chaos.

Choice between options: Instead of completely open-ended decisions (which overwhelm), practice choosing between two or three pre-determined options. "For lunch today, I'm choosing between Option A, Option B, or Option C." You have structure (only three options), flexibility (choosing between them), and reduced decision fatigue (not unlimited choices).

Script variations: Autistic individuals often feel comfortable when they know what to expect—like following a script. Cognitive flexibility practice involves creating multiple scripts for the same situation. What's your eating plan if you wake up late? What's your backup if your planned food isn't available? What's the alternative if you're more or less hungry than expected? Having multiple scripts ready reduces anxiety when circumstances change because you're still following a plan—just Plan B or C instead of Plan A.

Track successful variations: Keep a log of times when you varied your routine and nothing catastrophic happened. Your brain predicts disaster when you break rules. Showing your brain evidence that variation is safe gradually reduces that fear response. "I ate breakfast an hour late on Tuesday and was fine" becomes data that challenges the rule "breakfast must be at exactly 7:00 AM."

Elena, a 32-year-old autistic engineer, practiced cognitive flexibility by creating what she called "safe experiments." Each week, she identified one small rule to vary slightly in a controlled way. Week one: eat lunch 30 minutes later than usual. Week two: substitute one protein for another in dinner. Week three: eat a meal at a different location. She tracked each experiment: what she feared would happen, what actually happened, and how she felt afterward. Over six months, she accumulated evidence that small variations didn't cause disaster. This slowly weakened her eating disorder's hold on rigid rules. The pace was slow—much slower than standard eating disorder treatment expects. But it was effective because it matched her autistic brain's processing speed.

5.4 Structure Versus Restriction

This is the critical distinction. Some structure supports eating. Other structure restricts it. Learning the difference requires honest evaluation of your rules' actual effects.

Structure that helps has these characteristics:

- Supports consistent eating rather than limiting it

- Reduces decision fatigue and executive function demands
- Compensates for poor interoception or hunger cue difficulties
- Feels calming and organizing, not anxiety-provoking
- You can explain the rule's function without referencing weight, body size, or control

Examples: eating at regular times each day, using meal templates, having a rotation of acceptable foods, eating in consistent locations, following a general nutritional framework.

Restriction that harms has these characteristics:

- Results in eating less or with less variety
- Creates increasing anxiety and rigidity over time
- You can't articulate a logical reason for the rule beyond "it feels necessary"
- The rule keeps tightening (first no dessert on weekdays, then no dessert ever, then no foods with any added sugar)
- If the rule is broken, anxiety spikes dramatically and punitive responses follow
- The rule is primarily about control, body size, or weight rather than supporting eating

Examples: calorie limits, forbidden food categories without sensory justification, rigid timing that prevents eating if you're late, portion restrictions, rules about earning food through exercise.

The difficulty? Sometimes the same rule fits both categories depending on context and rigidity. Eating at scheduled times helps when it ensures you eat consistently despite poor hunger cues. It harms when you'd rather not eat if you miss the window by five minutes. Rotating between several breakfast options helps reduce decision fatigue. It harms when you can't eat breakfast at all if none of your rotation options are available.

Ask yourself these questions about each food rule:

1. Would I follow this rule if I didn't have an eating disorder?
2. Does this rule result in me eating adequately?
3. Can I be slightly flexible with this rule without intense anxiety?
4. Would a nutritionist without eating disorder training consider this rule reasonable?
5. Does this rule account for my autism, or is it just eating disorder control?

If you answer no to most of these questions, the rule likely serves restriction rather than structure. But don't try to eliminate all rules at once. That triggers chaos your autistic brain can't handle. Instead, gradually modify restrictive rules into supportive structure.

5.5 Special Interests as Recovery Assets

Special interests—the intense, focused interests common in autism—are typically viewed as a distraction or obsession to be managed. In eating disorder recovery, they're actually powerful tools (Grove et al., 2018).

Special interests provide:

Emotional regulation: When overwhelmed by eating disorder anxiety, engaging with your special interest reduces distress. It's not avoidance—it's using an inherent autism strength to regulate emotions. You need emotion regulation strategies that work with your autistic neurology, not against it.

Motivation and reward: Recovery requires sustained effort over long periods. Special interests can become reward systems. "After eating lunch, I spend 30 minutes engaging with my special interest." This isn't bribery—it's using natural motivation to support difficult behaviors.

Identity beyond the eating disorder: Eating disorders consume identity. "I'm anorexic" becomes your entire self-concept. Special interests remind you that you're a person with passions, expertise, and interests beyond the eating disorder. You're someone who loves astronomy, knows everything about trains, creates digital art, collects minerals. That identity supports recovery.

Structure and routine: Many special interests involve collecting, categorizing, or systematic engagement. These structured activities feel comfortable for autistic brains and can be scheduled as regular parts of your routine, providing predictability that supports overall regulation.

Social connection: Shared special interests create community. Online forums, local meetup groups, conventions—these spaces let you connect with others around genuine shared passion rather than forced socializing around eating disorder topics. Autistic-friendly social connection supports mental health, which supports eating disorder recovery.

Some therapists worry that special interests become escape from treatment. This happens occasionally—complete retreat into special interest while avoiding all recovery work. But more often, the problem is therapists not understanding how to harness special interests as recovery tools. The solution isn't limiting special interest time; it's strategically integrating special interests into recovery.

Raj, a 29-year-old autistic man with a special interest in astronomy, structured his recovery around his interest. His dietitian helped him create meal plans using space-themed names (Saturn Rings pasta, Moon Rock protein balls, Galaxy Smoothie). His therapist had him journal about recovery using astronomy metaphors. He rewarded eating disorder challenge behaviors with time working on his personal astronomy blog. He joined an astronomy club where he made friends without eating disorder talk dominating conversations. His special interest didn't distract from recovery—it facilitated recovery by providing motivation, structure, reward, and identity beyond illness. Standard treatment that viewed his astronomy interest as problematic avoidance had failed. Treatment that embraced and utilized his special interest succeeded.

5.6 Challenging Rules Strategically

You can't challenge all your eating disorder rules simultaneously. That's chaos. You need a strategic approach that identifies which rules to challenge first and how to challenge them effectively.

Rule prioritization: Create a list of all your food rules. Yes, write them down. Seeing them externalized often reveals how many you have. Then categorize them:

Priority 1 (challenge first): Rules actively causing malnutrition or health risk. Rules that prevent you from eating adequate calories, protein, or essential nutrients. These must be challenged even though they're scary.

Priority 2 (challenge soon): Rules that severely limit variety or create social isolation. Rules that mean you can't eat with family or friends. Rules that eliminate entire food categories without sensory justification.

Priority 3 (challenge eventually): Rules that create rigidity but don't immediately threaten health. Timing rules, location rules, order-of-eating rules. These can be addressed after more critical rules are challenged.

Priority 4 (possibly keep): Rules that genuinely support your autism without restricting. Eating at consistent times, using templates, having structure. These might be accommodations to maintain.

Start with one Priority 1 rule. Only one. Choose the rule that seems slightly less impossible than others in that category. If you can't eat any fats, maybe butter feels slightly less scary than oil. If you can't eat after 5 PM despite being hungry at 7 PM, maybe extending to 5:30 PM feels slightly more manageable than extending to 7 PM. Find your least impossible challenge and start there.

Rule modification process:

1. **Identify the rule's origin**: Where did this rule come from? Diet culture? Your eating disorder? A misunderstanding of nutrition? Knowing the rule's source helps challenge it. "Carbs are bad" came from diet culture misinformation, not from your autistic neurology needing that structure.
2. **Examine the rule's effects**: What actually happens when you follow this rule? Are you healthier? Or are you restricted, isolated, and struggling? Honest evaluation reveals that most eating disorder rules create harm, not benefit.
3. **Find evidence against the rule**: Research actual nutrition information. Talk to dietitians. Look at what healthy people actually eat. Gather evidence that contradicts your rule. "No eating after 7 PM" isn't based on metabolic science—it's arbitrary.
4. **Create a modification experiment**: Instead of completely abandoning the rule (too scary), modify it slightly. If the rule is "no carbs at dinner," try "one small carb serving at dinner." If the rule is "must exercise before eating," try "can eat even if I didn't exercise today once per week."
5. **Test and evaluate**: Follow the modified rule. Track what happens. Did catastrophe occur? Or did you survive? What did you learn? Use this data to further modify the rule.
6. **Gradually increase modification**: Over time, keep adjusting the rule toward greater flexibility and adequacy. Small steps repeatedly sustained create significant change eventually.

5.7 Creating Nourishing Routines

The goal isn't eliminating all routine—that would be impossible and undesirable for autistic brains. The goal is creating routines that nourish you physically and psychologically instead of restricting you.

Morning eating routines: Many autistic people struggle with morning transitions. Executive function is often poorest early in the day. Creating a simple morning eating routine that requires minimal decisions supports consistent breakfast. Example routine: Wake → bathroom → kitchen → choose from three pre-selected breakfast options → eat at table → brush teeth. Same sequence every morning. Predictable, manageable, ensures eating happens.

Meal preparation routines: Cooking is executive function hell—multiple steps, timing, decisions. Routinize what you can. Maybe Sunday is always meal prep day. Maybe you always prepare the same three dinner options each week. Maybe you use the same prep sequence: protein first, then starch, then vegetables. Routine removes decision points (Demetriou et al., 2018).

Eating environment routines: Eat in the same location when possible. Use the same dishes and utensils. Create sensory-friendly environment (comfortable lighting, minimal noise, pleasant temperature). Environmental consistency makes the sensory demands of eating itself more manageable.

Post-meal routines: What happens after eating affects your relationship with eating. If you immediately weigh yourself or scrutinize your body, you're reinforcing eating disorder behaviors. Instead, create post-meal routines that are calming and neutral: clean dishes, engage with special interest for 20 minutes, go for a gentle walk, read. These routines occupy the post-meal window when eating disorder thoughts often spike.

Flexibility intervals: Within your routine, schedule planned flexibility. Every few days, intentionally vary one element. Eat breakfast in a different location. Try a new snack. Eat dinner 30 minutes later. Scheduled flexibility prevents your routines from becoming eating disorder rigidity.

Sofia, a 26-year-old autistic woman, created what she called her "eating rhythm." Each day followed the same basic pattern, but with built-in variation points. Breakfast between 7:00-8:00 AM (timing flexibility). One of five breakfast options (choice flexibility). At her kitchen table (location consistency). Lunch at work between 12:00-1:00 PM (timing flexibility). Lunch from her prepared options (planning consistency). Dinner between 6:00-7:00 PM (timing flexibility). Dinner from rotation of seven options (variety within structure). Snacks at 10:00 AM and 3:00 PM (timing consistency). This rhythm provided enough structure to support her autistic need for routine while building enough flexibility to prevent eating disorder rigidity.

5.8 Core Concepts Recap

Autistic pattern-based thinking is a strength that eating disorders exploit. Your brain's natural preference for rules, routines, and structure makes you vulnerable to rigid eating disorder thinking. But with strategic approaches, you can maintain enough structure to support your autistic neurology while developing enough flexibility to eat adequately in various circumstances.

The work isn't eliminating all food rules or becoming completely spontaneous—that doesn't match autistic cognition and sets you up for failure. The work is distinguishing helpful structure from harmful restriction, gradually building cognitive flexibility within structured frameworks, strategically challenging rules that actively harm you, and creating nourishing routines that support consistent eating without feeding eating disorder rigidity.

Use your special interests as recovery tools, not distractions. Build middle-ground thinking to escape all-or-nothing traps. Develop graduated flexibility that respects your autism while preventing eating disorder control. Challenge rules systematically rather than chaotically. And remember: adequate nutrition with structure that works for your autistic brain is recovery. Perfect flexibility isn't required.

Chapter 6.0: Reconnecting with Interoception

Your body sends signals all day long. Hungry. Full. Thirsty. Need the bathroom. Heart racing. Breathing shallow. Most people process these signals automatically without conscious effort. But for many autistic individuals, these internal body signals arrive scrambled, delayed, or don't arrive at all. This is **interoception**—the sense that tells you what's happening inside your body—and when it's impaired, eating becomes a cognitive puzzle rather than a natural response to physical need.

This chapter teaches you to work with poor interoception instead of fighting against it. You'll learn alternative strategies for knowing when your body needs food, how to distinguish physical hunger from emotional needs, and how to build enough body trust to support consistent eating despite unreliable signals.

6.1 Understanding Interoceptive Difficulties

Interoception is your eighth sense—the one nobody talks about in elementary school. While you learn about sight, hearing, touch, taste, and smell, interoception quietly operates in the background, monitoring your internal state. It tells you when your heart is pounding from anxiety, when your bladder is full, when you're getting overheated, when you're hungry, when you're comfortably full (Garfinkel et al., 2015).

Research shows that approximately 70% of autistic adults experience interoception difficulties (DuBois et al., 2016). That's not a small subset—that's the majority. For autistic women with eating disorders, poor interoception creates a particularly challenging situation. You're supposed to recover by "listening to your body" when your body isn't speaking clearly.

Interoception difficulties manifest differently for different people. Some autistic individuals experience **low interoceptive awareness**—they genuinely don't feel hunger signals until they're extremely hungry, don't notice fullness until they're uncomfortably overfull, don't detect thirst until they're dehydrated. The signals might be there, but they're not reaching conscious awareness (Garfinkel et al., 2015).

Others experience **interoceptive confusion**—they feel sensations but can't identify what they mean. Is that uncomfortable feeling in your stomach hunger, nausea, anxiety, or fullness? All of these produce similar physical sensations, and your brain struggles to differentiate them. This confusion makes appropriate responses nearly impossible. You might eat when you're anxious (not hungry), or skip meals when you're actually starving (because you misread the signal as something else).

Still others experience **delayed interoception**—signals arrive hours after they should. You don't feel hungry at breakfast time, then suddenly at 3 PM you're ravenously hungry and shaky. Or you eat a normal meal and don't feel full until two hours later when the discomfort finally registers. This delay throws off normal eating patterns and makes portion regulation extremely difficult.

Brain imaging research helps explain why this happens. Studies show that autistic individuals process interoceptive information differently, with altered activation in brain regions responsible for integrating internal body signals—particularly the insula and anterior cingulate cortex (Quattrocki & Friston, 2014). This isn't psychological. It's neurological. Your nervous system genuinely processes internal signals differently than neurotypical nervous systems.

Think about what this means for eating disorder recovery. Standard treatment tells you to eat when you're hungry and stop when you're full. But if you can't reliably detect hunger or fullness, following this guidance is impossible. You're being asked to navigate using instruments that don't function properly. No wonder recovery feels so difficult.

6.2 Alternative Navigation Methods

If your internal signals don't work reliably, you need external frameworks. This isn't giving up on recovery—it's adapting recovery to match your neurology.

Time-based eating: Instead of waiting for hunger signals that might not arrive, eat based on time intervals. Most bodies need food every 3-4 hours. Create a schedule: breakfast within an hour of waking, snack mid-morning, lunch midday, afternoon snack, dinner in evening, evening snack if needed. You're not eating because you feel hungry—you're eating because it's time to eat and your body needs fuel (Mehling et al., 2018).

This isn't eating disorder rigidity if the schedule serves nutrition. The difference is that time-based eating ensures adequate intake, while eating disorder time rules restrict intake. Eating disorder rule: "I can only eat between 12 PM and 6 PM." Time-based eating: "I eat roughly every 3-4 hours to ensure my body gets energy throughout the day."

Energy level monitoring: While you might not feel hunger clearly, you probably notice energy drops. Do you get shaky, lightheaded, irritable, or tired? These are hunger manifestations your body might signal more clearly than stomach sensations. Learn your pattern. If you consistently get irritable around 11 AM, that's your body saying it needs food, even if your stomach isn't growling. If you crash at 3 PM, that's a signal. Honor these indirect hunger cues.

Cognitive tracking: Keep a simple eating log—not to restrict, but to identify patterns. Note when you eat, what you eat, and how you feel physically and mentally at various times. Over weeks, patterns emerge. Maybe you function better with four smaller meals than three large ones. Maybe you need a substantial breakfast even though you never feel hungry in the morning. The data reveals what your interoception can't tell you directly.

Environmental cues: Use external reminders. Phone alarms for meal times. Calendar notifications. Ask trusted people to remind you. These aren't crutches—they're accommodations for a neurological difference. Someone with vision impairment uses glasses. You use external cues to compensate for internal signal impairment.

Portion guides: Since fullness signals are unreliable, use external guides for appropriate portions. Your dietitian can help determine adequate serving sizes. Use measuring tools initially to learn what appropriate portions look like. This isn't eating disorder measuring—it's learning portion awareness when internal fullness cues don't guide you. Eventually, you might develop visual estimation skills, but external guides provide initial structure.

Maria, a 28-year-old autistic accountant, spent years trying to eat intuitively based on hunger and fullness. It never worked. She'd skip breakfast because she didn't feel hungry, work through lunch absorbed in projects, then binge at dinner because she was starving. Her therapist kept encouraging her to "get more in touch with her body." After her autism diagnosis, a new approach emerged: structured eating times regardless of hunger signals. Breakfast at 7:30 AM (never feels hungry but eats anyway), snack at 10:30 AM, lunch at 1:00 PM, snack at 4:00 PM, dinner at 7:00 PM. Within three months, her eating stabilized. She still rarely felt clear hunger, but her body got consistent nutrition. Six months later, she started noticing subtle hunger signals she'd never recognized before—possibly because consistent eating helped her nervous system regulate better. But even with improved interoception, she maintained time-based structure as her primary framework.

6.3 Improving Interoceptive Awareness

Poor interoception isn't completely fixed, but it can improve somewhat with deliberate practice. The key is patience and realistic expectations. You're not aiming for perfect internal awareness—you're aiming for slightly better recognition of some signals some of the time.

Body scan practices: Adapted mindfulness techniques can help increase interoceptive awareness. Several times daily, pause and systematically notice sensations in different body parts. Not interpreting or judging—just noticing. Do you feel tension anywhere? Warmth or coolness? Pressure? Emptiness? Fullness? This practice strengthens the neural pathways between body sensations and conscious awareness (Mehling et al., 2018).

Start very brief—30 seconds. Longer body scans overwhelm if you're not used to interoceptive focus. Gradually extend as you build tolerance. Some autistic individuals find body scans activate anxiety rather than awareness. If this is you, skip this technique and use others instead.

Hunger scale practice: Create a simple hunger scale: 1 (extremely hungry, shaky, lightheaded), 3 (moderately hungry, ready to eat), 5 (neutral, neither hungry nor full), 7 (comfortably satisfied), 10 (uncomfortably overfull, physical discomfort). Several times daily, pause and ask: where am I on this scale right now?

Initially, you might have no idea. That's okay. Make your best guess. Over time, with repeated practice and comparison to external factors (time since last meal, energy levels, physical sensations), your accuracy improves. You're training your brain to notice and categorize interoceptive information (Herbert & Pollatos, 2012).

Eating speed awareness: Eating slowly gives interoception time to register. Fullness signals take 15-20 minutes to travel from stomach to brain (Horner et al., 2011). If you eat quickly, you overshoot fullness before the signal arrives. Practice eating at a pace that allows signal processing: put utensils down between bites, chew thoroughly, pause mid-meal to assess how you feel.

For autistic individuals who eat for sensory regulation (the chewing motion, the taste, the routine), slowing down feels uncomfortable. Balance is needed. Maybe eat slowly enough to allow some fullness awareness but not so slowly it feels torturous. Some meals can be slower (low-stress environments) while others are faster (high-demand days). Recovery doesn't require perfection.

Hunger priming: Before eating, deliberately focus on physical sensations for 30 seconds. Notice your stomach, your energy level, any sensations you might associate with hunger. This priming tells your brain "pay attention to hunger-related signals now." After eating, repeat the process, focusing on sensations of fullness or satisfaction. You're teaching your nervous system to prioritize these particular interoceptive signals.

6.4 Physical Hunger Versus Emotional Needs

Here's where interoception difficulties create confusion. Physical hunger and emotional distress produce overlapping physical sensations. Both can create stomach discomfort, tension, agitation, and urgency. Without clear interoceptive discrimination, you might eat when you're actually anxious, or ignore hunger thinking it's just anxiety (Kitayama et al., 2000).

Physical hunger characteristics: Typically builds gradually over hours since last eating, produces emptiness or growling in stomach, improves after eating any food (not specific foods), includes physical symptoms like low energy or lightheadedness, timing correlates with last meal (3-4 hours typically).

Emotional hunger characteristics: Comes on suddenly regardless of when you last ate, produces tension or discomfort but not stomach emptiness, seeks specific comfort foods rather than any food, includes mental symptoms like urgency or intrusive thoughts about food, timing correlates with stress or emotional triggers rather than eating schedule (Macht, 2008).

The problem? These categories aren't always distinct. Anxiety can produce genuine stomach sensations that feel identical to hunger. Hunger can trigger emotional distress that then confuses the signal further. And alexithymia—difficulty identifying emotions, which affects about 50% of autistic adults (Bird & Cook, 2013)—means you might not even recognize what emotion you're experiencing to know it's emotional hunger.

Practical differentiation strategies:

Time check: When did you last eat? If it's been 4+ hours, probably physical hunger regardless of what it feels like. If you ate 30 minutes ago, probably not physical hunger even if your stomach feels uncomfortable.

Food type test: Physical hunger accepts any food. Emotional hunger wants specific foods, usually comfort foods or foods associated with restriction. Ask yourself: would I eat raw vegetables right now? If yes, probably physical hunger. If you only want specific foods, might be emotional eating (though autistic sensory needs complicate this test—sometimes you genuinely can only eat specific foods due to sensory issues, not emotions).

Intensity pattern: Physical hunger builds gradually. Emotional hunger feels sudden and urgent. If the hunger sensation appeared within five minutes, it's probably emotional or anxiety-driven rather than true physical need.

Post-eating evaluation: Eat something. If the discomfort resolves, it was physical hunger. If eating doesn't resolve the uncomfortable feeling, you were likely addressing an emotional need with food, which doesn't actually resolve that need.

Layla, a 31-year-old autistic graphic designer, struggled to distinguish hunger from anxiety for years. Both produced similar stomach sensations. Her therapist taught her a simple algorithm: Check time since last meal. If less than 3 hours, not hungry—anxiety. If more than 3 hours, eat regardless of what it feels like. If more than 3 hours and she just ate but still feels "hungry," not hungry—anxiety. This external framework bypassed her interoception difficulties entirely. Was it perfect? No. Sometimes she ate when she wasn't truly hungry, and sometimes she didn't eat when she was slightly hungry but within the 3-hour window. But it was functional. Her nutrition improved dramatically. After a year of consistent eating using this framework, her interoception improved enough that she could sometimes actually feel the difference between hunger and anxiety. But the framework remained her primary tool.

6.5 Sensory Discomfort and Fullness

This distinction matters enormously for autistic women with eating disorders. Sensory discomfort from eating and dangerous fullness feel similar but require different responses.

Sensory discomfort happens when food triggers sensory processing issues. The texture felt wrong, the temperature was off, you ate too quickly and the sensory input overwhelmed you, the food's smell lingers and bothers you. Your stomach might feel uncomfortable, but you're not medically overfull—you're sensorially overwhelmed by the eating experience (Cermak et al., 2010).

Dangerous fullness happens when you've eaten significantly beyond your body's capacity. Your stomach is stretched beyond comfortable limits, you feel physically ill, movement is difficult, genuine nausea occurs. This requires medical attention if severe and indicates you need to adjust portion sizes or eating speed.

Many autistic women interpret sensory discomfort as dangerous fullness, then restrict to avoid that feeling. The eating disorder hijacks legitimate sensory distress to justify restriction. "I ate too much, I feel terrible" actually means "the sensory experience of eating overwhelmed me, and now I feel uncomfortable." The solution isn't eating less—it's managing sensory demands differently.

Distinguishing factors:

Quantity check: How much did you actually eat? Compare to standard portions. If you ate a normal meal (not objectively excessive), discomfort is probably sensory, not overfullness. If you ate significantly more than a typical meal, might be genuine overfullness.

Sensation location: Sensory discomfort often involves more than stomach—tension throughout body, sensory overwhelm in other systems (sounds too loud, lights too bright), general dysregulation. Dangerous fullness centers primarily on stomach distension and nausea.

Relief methods: Sensory discomfort improves with sensory regulation strategies (quiet space, dim lights, weighted blanket, time to decompress). Dangerous fullness only improves with time for digestion and won't improve from sensory accommodations.

Pattern recognition: Does this happen every time you eat, regardless of portion size? Probably sensory. Does it only happen when you eat significantly more than usual? Probably genuine overfullness.

Accommodation strategies for sensory eating discomfort:

Eat in sensory-friendly environments (quiet, comfortable lighting, minimal distractions). Eat slowly to reduce sensory overwhelm from rapid food input. Choose foods with acceptable sensory properties when possible. Plan post-meal regulation time (don't schedule demanding activities immediately after eating). Use sensory tools after eating (weighted blanket, gentle movement, engaging with special interests).

Most importantly: don't let eating disorders use sensory discomfort to justify restriction. Yes, eating sometimes feels uncomfortable due to sensory processing. That doesn't mean you should eat less—it means you need better sensory support around eating.

6.6 Building Body Trust

This is the hardest part. How do you trust your body when your body's signals are unreliable? The answer: you don't fully trust your body. You build a hybrid system of partial body trust plus external supports.

Trust what you can trust: Maybe your body signals extreme hunger reliably even if subtle hunger goes unnoticed. Trust those extreme signals. Maybe your body signals dangerous fullness even if comfortable satiation is unclear. Trust those signals. Identify which interoceptive signals you can somewhat rely on, and honor those while using external frameworks for the unclear signals (Jenkinson et al., 2018).

Trust the pattern, not individual instances: Your body might not signal hunger reliably on Tuesday morning. But the pattern over weeks shows you consistently function better eating breakfast. Trust the pattern over the unreliable daily signal. You're building trust through data collection, not through blind faith in moment-to-moment sensations.

Trust structure: This sounds contradictory to body trust, but it's not. Trusting structure (meal schedules, portion guides, external cues) is trusting that your body needs regular fuel even when it doesn't tell you so clearly. You're trusting your body's metabolic needs instead of trusting your body's signal system.

Gradual trust experiments: Occasionally test your interoception. Skip setting a meal alarm one day and see if you notice hunger signals. Vary portion sizes slightly and notice if fullness awareness changes. These experiments gather information about your interoception's current accuracy without abandoning all structure. If experiments consistently show your signals remain unreliable, that's valuable information—you need continued external support.

Separate body trust from eating disorder fear: Eating disorders masquerade as body wisdom. "My body doesn't want breakfast" might be your eating disorder restricting, not your body communicating real needs. True body trust means trusting your body's actual needs—regular fuel, adequate nutrition, variety for health—not trusting eating disorder thoughts disguised as body signals.

Chen, a 33-year-old autistic researcher, spent two years working on body trust. Early in recovery, he used complete external structure—alarms for every meal, measured portions, cognitive tracking. He didn't trust his body at all because his body had never signaled hunger clearly. After a year of consistent eating, his therapist suggested small trust experiments. One day per week, Chen turned off meal alarms and tried eating when he felt hungry. Initially, he'd forget meals entirely. But after months of experiments, patterns emerged. He could sometimes notice hunger if he paid deliberate attention. He could usually notice extreme hunger. He rarely noticed comfortable fullness. Based on these experiments, Chen built a hybrid system: time-based structure for most meals (because hunger signals remained unreliable), but permission to eat earlier if extreme hunger appeared (because that signal he could trust), and external portion guides since fullness awareness stayed unclear. This wasn't perfect body trust. It was realistic trust in a body with interoception differences.

6.7 Your Takeaways

Poor interoception makes eating disorder recovery significantly harder when treatment assumes reliable internal signals. For autistic women, recovery requires adapted approaches that work with interoceptive difficulties rather than pretending they don't exist.

You need external frameworks—time-based eating, portion guides, energy monitoring—to replace unreliable internal signals. These aren't eating disorder rules if they support adequate nutrition. They're accommodations for neurological differences.

Interoception can improve somewhat with practice, but don't expect dramatic changes. You're aiming for slightly better awareness, not perfect internal sensing. Meanwhile, maintain external supports that ensure consistent nutrition regardless of signal clarity.

Learn to distinguish physical hunger from emotional needs using external criteria (time since last meal, pattern recognition) since interoceptive discrimination is difficult. Recognize that sensory discomfort from eating isn't the same as dangerous fullness, though they feel similar.

Build realistic body trust—a hybrid of trusting signals you can somewhat rely on while using external supports for unclear signals. Trust the patterns and structure that support adequate nutrition even when moment-to-moment signals are confusing.

Recovery with poor interoception is absolutely possible. It looks different from neurotypical recovery. It involves more external structure, more cognitive work, and more patience with yourself. But thousands of autistic individuals maintain recovery using these adapted approaches. You can too.

Chapter 7.0: Emotional Recovery Strategies

Emotions. For many autistic individuals, they're confusing, overwhelming, and difficult to manage. You might not know what you're feeling until the emotion has passed. Or you feel everything intensely without ability to modulate. Or you go numb and feel nothing at all. When eating disorders enter this picture, food becomes the primary emotion regulation tool—restriction numbs feelings, bingeing soothes distress, purging releases tension. Taking away those coping mechanisms without providing alternatives leaves you defenseless against emotional overwhelm.

This chapter teaches emotion regulation strategies that work with autistic neurology. You'll learn to process feelings without numbing through food control, use stimming and special interests therapeutically, manage meltdowns and shutdowns without turning to eating disorder behaviors, and develop self-compassion for your authentic, autistic self.

7.1 When You Cannot Name Feelings

Alexithymia—literally "no words for feelings"—describes difficulty identifying and describing emotions. About 50% of autistic adults experience significant alexithymia compared to 10% of the general population (Bird & Cook, 2013). You know you feel bad, but you can't name the specific emotion. Is this sadness? Anxiety? Frustration? Loneliness? All emotions blend into generic "bad feeling" or "good feeling."

For eating disorder recovery, alexithymia creates serious complications. Traditional therapy asks you to identify emotional triggers for eating disorder behaviors. "What were you feeling right before you restricted?" But if you can't identify what you were feeling, you can't answer. Therapists might interpret this as resistance when actually it's alexithymia—a neurological difference in emotional processing (Kinnaird et al., 2019).

Alexithymia also makes it nearly impossible to distinguish physical hunger from emotional needs, as we discussed in section 6.4. If you can't identify emotions clearly, how do you know if that uncomfortable feeling is hunger, anxiety, sadness, or boredom? You might restrict because you think you're not hungry when actually you're anxious about an upcoming meeting. Or binge because you think you're hungry when actually you're lonely and seeking comfort.

Strategies for working with alexithymia:

Simplified emotion categories: Forget nuanced emotion identification. Use simple categories: Good, Bad, Neutral. Some people add two more: Very Bad, Very Good. That's it. You don't need to distinguish between disappointment, frustration, and sadness. They're all "Bad." This isn't emotionally sophisticated, but it's functional. Once you identify the general category, you can respond appropriately without needing specific labels (Samson et al., 2012).

Physical sensation mapping: Alexithymia doesn't mean you don't feel emotions physically—it means you can't label them. Map physical sensations instead. Maybe tension in your shoulders happens with certain emotions. Stomach butterflies with others. Heaviness in your chest with still others. Create a personal sensation map. You might not know these sensations mean "anxiety" or "sadness," but you know "shoulder tension feeling" or "heavy chest feeling." That's enough to identify patterns and respond.

Contextual emotion identification: Use external context instead of internal awareness. If someone just criticized you, you're probably upset even if you can't feel it clearly. If you're about to give a presentation, you're probably nervous. If a friend canceled plans, you're probably disappointed. Context provides emotion labels when interoception can't.

Behavioral indicators: How are you acting? Eating disorder behaviors often reveal emotions you can't consciously identify. Restricting might indicate anxiety or desire for control. Bingeing might indicate loneliness, boredom, or overwhelm. Purging might indicate self-hatred or need to release tension. Your behaviors communicate emotions your conscious mind doesn't recognize. Working with a therapist to identify these behavior-emotion links helps you understand yourself better.

Emotion wheels and charts: Visual tools help some people. Emotion wheels show different emotions with related physical sensations and facial expressions. When you feel bad, reference the wheel. Which facial expression matches yours? Which physical sensations are you experiencing? This external framework provides labels your internal processing doesn't generate naturally (Kinnaird et al., 2019).

Priya, a 29-year-old autistic social worker, experienced severe alexithymia. Her therapist would ask "What were you feeling before you binged?" Priya had no idea. She felt "something bad" but couldn't specify further. Traditional emotion-focused therapy wasn't working. They shifted to a simpler system. Good, Bad, Very Bad. When Priya felt Bad or Very Bad, she'd check: Have I eaten in the past 4 hours? If no, eat first—might be hunger masquerading as emotion. If yes, use a non-food coping strategy from her list. What strategy? She'd check her physical sensations. Tension? Do progressive muscle relaxation. Restless energy? Walk or stim. Mental overwhelm? Engage with special interest. This system worked. She never developed sophisticated emotion identification, but she didn't need to. Behavioral responses based on simple categorization and physical sensations achieved the same result—managing distress without eating disorder behaviors.

7.2 Meltdowns Shutdowns and Eating

Autistic meltdowns and shutdowns are stress responses to overwhelming experiences—too much sensory input, too many social demands, too much emotional intensity, accumulated stress without recovery time (Mazefsky et al., 2013). Neither is voluntary. Both are your nervous system's way of attempting to protect itself from overload.

Meltdowns involve outward explosive responses: crying, screaming, physical aggression toward objects or self, intense emotional expression. You lose ability to regulate behavior and responses. Afterward, you feel exhausted, ashamed, and often confused about what triggered such intense reaction.

Shutdowns involve inward collapse: going nonverbal or minimally verbal, withdrawing completely, inability to process information, feeling numb or disconnected. You can't engage with others or your environment. Afterward, you need significant recovery time before functioning normally.

Eating disorders interact with meltdowns and shutdowns in several ways. First, malnutrition and inconsistent eating increase meltdown and shutdown frequency. Your nervous system is already stressed from inadequate nutrition. Any additional stressor pushes you over the edge more easily. Second, eating disorder behaviors sometimes serve as maladaptive attempts to prevent or manage meltdowns and shutdowns. Restriction numbs emotions that might trigger meltdowns. Bingeing soothes and distracts from overload. Purging releases built-up tension before it explodes into meltdown.

Third, meltdowns and shutdowns themselves trigger eating disorder behaviors. After a meltdown, shame and distress drive restriction as punishment or compensation. After shutdown, returning to baseline requires self-soothing, which might involve bingeing. The cycle perpetuates itself: inadequate nutrition increases autistic stress responses, which trigger eating disorder behaviors, which worsen nutrition, which increases stress responses further (Kinnaird et al., 2019).

Breaking the cycle:

Adequate nutrition reduces frequency: As we've discussed throughout this book, consistent eating stabilizes your nervous system. It doesn't eliminate meltdowns and shutdowns—you're autistic, stress responses will still happen—but it raises your threshold. Stressors that previously triggered meltdowns might become manageable. This alone is powerful reason to maintain recovery eating.

Early warning recognition: Meltdowns and shutdowns build over time, though the final trigger might seem sudden. Learn your early warning signs. Maybe you get snappish or irritable hours before meltdown. Maybe you start withdrawing or having trouble concentrating before shutdown. Catching early warnings allows preventive intervention—remove yourself from stressors, use regulation strategies, rest—before full meltdown or shutdown occurs (Mazefsky et al., 2013).

Preventive scheduling: If you know certain situations trigger meltdowns or shutdowns, limit exposure or schedule recovery time after. Don't stack stressors. If you have a demanding work meeting, don't schedule social obligations the same evening. Build in decompression time. Your eating disorder might protest this accommodation—it wants you busy and stressed so it can offer "help" through restriction or other behaviors. Ignore the eating disorder. Prevent overload proactively.

Meltdown and shutdown protocols: Create simple plans for what to do during and after these events that don't involve eating disorder behaviors. During meltdown: safe space, sensory tools, time alone, no demands for social interaction or problem-solving. After meltdown: rest, gentle sensory regulation, no self-criticism. During shutdown: minimal interaction, safe quiet space, permission to be nonverbal, basic physical care only. After shutdown: slow return to activities, extended recovery time, self-compassion. These protocols provide alternatives to eating disorder responses.

Separate eating from stress responses: Make it a rule: no eating disorder behaviors for 24 hours after meltdown or shutdown. Your brain is dysregulated and makes poor decisions post-crisis. Restriction as self-punishment or bingeing as self-soothing might feel compelling, but they don't actually help—they complicate recovery and feed the cycle. Stick to your structured meal plan regardless of meltdowns or shutdowns. Eating stays consistent even when everything else feels chaotic.

7.3 Processing Without Numbing

Eating disorder restriction numbs emotion effectively. When you're malnourished, emotions dull. Everything feels flat. For autistic individuals who experience emotions intensely or confusingly, this numbness feels like relief. The problem: it's not selective numbness. You don't just numb pain—you numb everything. Joy, connection, passion, motivation. Everything disappears into gray fog.

Recovery means feeling again. Scary prospect. How do you process intense, confusing emotions without numbing through restriction?

Create emotional intensity tolerance gradually: You don't go from numbed to feeling everything fully immediately. That's overwhelming. Build tolerance slowly. Set aside small amounts of time—10 minutes initially—to feel emotions without attempting to numb. Notice what comes up. Don't judge, just observe. After 10 minutes, use a regulation strategy or engage with something neutral. Gradually extend these "feeling windows" as tolerance increases. You're building emotional muscles that atrophied during eating disorder numbness.

External processing through structure: Autistic brains often process better through external structure than internal reflection. Journal feelings using templates ("Today I felt [emotion] when [situation]. My body felt [physical sensation]. I coped by [action]."). Talk through feelings with trusted person using structured format. Create diagrams or mind maps of emotional situations. The structure makes the amorphous mess of feelings more manageable (Samson et al., 2012).

Movement for emotion release: Intense emotions need physical release. Autistic individuals often regulate better through movement than through verbal processing. Walk, run, dance, bounce on a trampoline, do repetitive physical activities. Movement releases emotional tension without requiring verbal processing or emotional sophistication. It works even with alexithymia—you don't need to name what you're feeling to move until the intensity decreases.

Special interests as emotional refuge: When emotions overwhelm, engaging with special interests provides regulated escape without numbing through restriction. This isn't avoidance—it's legitimate regulation. You need breaks from emotional intensity. Special interests offer those breaks while maintaining engagement with life. Restriction offers breaks by disconnecting you from life entirely. Very different outcomes.

Permission for emotional inefficiency: Neurotypical people process emotions relatively quickly and move on. Autistic emotional processing often takes longer and feels less efficient. You might need to process the same situation multiple times over several days. That's okay. Recovery doesn't require neurotypical emotional processing speed. It requires finding ways to process that work for you, at whatever pace that takes.

Aisha, a 26-year-old autistic nurse, used restriction to numb overwhelming emotions for years. Early recovery felt unbearable—emotions she'd suppressed for years came flooding back. Her therapist taught her graduated emotion exposure. Week one: allow yourself to feel for five minutes daily, then engage with special interest (Islamic art history). Week two: extend to 10 minutes. By month three, Aisha could tolerate emotional experiences for extended periods without overwhelming panic. She developed an emotional processing routine: journal using a template her therapist created, go for a run, process more while running, come home and engage with art history research for an hour. This combination of structured processing, movement, and special interest engagement worked better than traditional talk therapy had. Her emotions no longer felt like enemies requiring numbing through restriction. They felt like information she could process using her personal toolkit.

7.4 Stimming and Healthy Coping

Stimming—self-stimulatory behavior—includes repetitive movements or sounds that provide sensory input and regulation. Rocking, hand-flapping, pacing, humming, repeating words or phrases, touching textures, spinning objects. For autistic individuals, stimming is natural self-regulation (Kapp et al., 2019).

Many autistic women mask their stims—suppress them in public because they've been told stimming is inappropriate, weird, or childish. This suppression requires constant energy and increases baseline stress. You're essentially preventing your nervous system from regulating naturally, which means external stressors hit you harder and recovery from stress takes longer.

Eating disorders sometimes function as socially acceptable stims. Restriction creates physical sensation (hunger, emptiness) that provides constant sensory input. Bingeing provides oral stimulation and intense sensory experience. Purging creates strong physical sensation. Over-exercising provides proprioceptive input and repetitive movement. These aren't healthy stims—they harm your body—but they serve similar regulatory functions as natural stims.

Recovery requires reclaiming healthy stimming as legitimate regulation strategy.

Identify your natural stims: What did you do as a child before anyone told you to stop? What do you do when alone that you suppress in public? These are your authentic stims. They're not shameful or wrong—they're your nervous system's natural regulation tools. Reclaim them.

Find socially acceptable stims: If you need to stim in public but feel self-conscious, identify subtle stims that don't draw attention. Fidget tools, clicking pens, tapping rhythms with fingers, chewing gum, wearing textured clothing you can touch discretely. These provide regulation without obvious visibility. The goal isn't hiding autism forever—it's giving you options for when public stimming feels unsafe while working toward broader acceptance of visible stims.

Stim breaks: Just like smokers take smoke breaks, you need stim breaks. Step away from demands, engage with your stims for five minutes, return regulated. This prevents buildup of stress that might otherwise trigger eating disorder behaviors. Your employer doesn't need to know you're stimming specifically—just that you need brief movement or sensory breaks periodically.

Connect stimming to eating disorder urges: Notice the link between stim suppression and eating disorder urges. Many autistic women find that after a day of suppressing stims (meetings, social events, professional settings), eating disorder behaviors intensify. You need regulation. If healthy regulation (stimming) wasn't available, unhealthy regulation (eating disorder behaviors) becomes appealing. The solution: stim more, restrict less. Allow stim breaks during stressful days. Stim freely at home. Give your nervous system the regulation it needs through healthy means (Kapp et al., 2019).

Stimming during meals: For some autistic individuals, eating is dysregulating—sitting still, focusing on internal sensations, processing sensory input from food. Allowing gentle stimming during meals helps. Rock slightly in your chair, fidget with a stim tool with your non-eating hand, hum quietly if you're alone. This isn't disordered eating—it's autistic regulation that makes eating possible.

7.5 Managing Overwhelm Differently

Overwhelm is the autistic experience of having your processing capacity exceeded by demands. Too much sensory input, too many decisions, too much social interaction, too many changes, accumulated stress without rest. When overwhelmed, you can't think clearly, regulate emotions, or make good decisions (Mazefsky et al., 2013).

Eating disorders offer apparent overwhelm management. Restriction simplifies life—fewer decisions about food, less social eating, diminished emotional capacity. Bingeing and purging provide intense focus that temporarily blocks out overwhelming stimuli. Over-exercising creates controlled, predictable activity when everything else feels chaotic. These strategies work short-term. They fail long-term because they add health complications and life restriction that ultimately create more overwhelm.

Legitimate overwhelm management strategies:

Reduce demands proactively: You have limited processing capacity. When you exceed it, you pay the price through meltdowns, shutdowns, or eating disorder behaviors. The solution isn't pushing through—it's reducing demands to manageable levels. Say no to optional obligations. Simplify your schedule. Eliminate unnecessary complexity from daily life. Your eating disorder might claim this is weakness or laziness. It's not. It's appropriate accommodation for your neurology.

Environmental control: Change your environment to reduce sensory overwhelm. Dim lights, wear noise-canceling headphones, control temperature, minimize visual clutter, avoid strong smells. These changes reduce baseline stress, which increases capacity for other demands. You're not being oversensitive—you're managing your sensory processing differences appropriately.

Predictability and routine: As we discussed in section 5.7, routine reduces cognitive load. When your day follows predictable patterns, you use less processing capacity on logistics and have more available for unexpected challenges. Eating disorders exploit this by offering rigid routines. The difference: eating disorder routines restrict life. Healthy routines support life. Choose routines that enable adequate eating and functioning, not routines that limit them (Hollocks et al., 2019).

Regular recovery time: Autistic nervous systems need more recovery time than neurotypical ones. Social interaction, sensory-intense environments, unpredictable situations, masking—all require recovery time. Schedule it deliberately. Time alone, engaging in special interests, minimal demands, sensory-friendly environment. This isn't optional self-care—it's mandatory nervous system maintenance. Without it, overwhelm accumulates until you can't function.

Externalize decisions: Decision fatigue contributes heavily to overwhelm. Reduce decisions wherever possible. Meal planning templates (section 4.6), clothing capsule wardrobes, simplified routines—all eliminate unnecessary decisions and preserve processing capacity for important things. Eating disorders offer to make eating decisions for you through rules. Better solution: create decision frameworks that ensure adequate nutrition without eating disorder control.

Marcus, a 34-year-old autistic software developer, lived in chronic overwhelm before understanding autistic nervous system needs. His coping strategy: restrict eating to create numbness and simplification. Recovery required completely restructuring his life for overwhelm prevention. He simplified his apartment (minimal visual clutter), created extensive routines (same clothes combinations, same meal rotations, same weekly schedule), negotiated remote work (eliminated commute and office sensory demands), and scheduled mandatory recovery time (two hours nightly of special interest engagement, no social obligations on weekends). These changes felt self-indulgent initially. But within three months, his baseline stress decreased dramatically. Eating disorder urges diminished because he wasn't using restriction to manage constant overwhelm anymore. The overwhelm itself decreased through appropriate accommodations.

7.6 Routine and Emotional Stability

Predictability calms autistic nervous systems. Routine provides that predictability. Research shows that autistic individuals experience less anxiety and better emotional regulation when daily life follows consistent patterns (Hollocks et al., 2019). This isn't pathological rigidity—it's adaptive use of routine to reduce processing demands and emotional volatility.

Eating disorders co-opt this need for routine. They offer extremely rigid patterns that reduce anxiety through complete control. The problem: these patterns also restrict life, health, and functioning. Recovery requires maintaining enough routine to support emotional stability without falling into eating disorder rigidity.

Routine for emotional regulation: Create consistent daily structure that includes time for regulation activities. Morning routine might include stimming time, engaging with special interest, predictable breakfast. Evening routine might include decompression, sensory-friendly activities, consistent sleep schedule. These routines bookend your day with regulation, making the middle part more manageable.

Mealtime routines: As discussed in section 4.5, structured mealtimes support consistent eating for autistic individuals. But they also support emotional stability by providing predictable self-care. You know you'll be nourished at specific intervals. You know what to expect. This predictability reduces anxiety and frees mental energy for other aspects of life.

Transition routines: Transitions between activities are difficult for many autistic people. Creating small routines around transitions helps. Five minutes of stimming before moving to the next activity, brief special interest engagement, predictable sequence of actions. These transition routines make change more manageable and reduce the emotional dysregulation that often accompanies transitions.

Flexibility within routine: Remember from section 5.3, you need graduated flexibility practice. Build slight variations into your routines to prevent them from becoming eating disorder rigidity. Maybe Tuesday's morning routine includes five minutes of something different. Maybe Friday evening routine varies slightly.

Enough flexibility to prevent rigidity, enough routine to provide stability.

Emergency deviation plans: Sometimes routine breaks—travel, illness, unexpected events. Having pre-planned emergency protocols reduces the emotional crisis these disruptions create. "When routine breaks, I follow Emergency Plan A: simplified eating (safe foods, structured times), maximum sensory accommodation, minimal social demands, extended recovery time." Knowing you have a plan makes routine disruptions less terrifying.

7.7 Self Compassion for Authentic You

This might be the hardest work in recovery: accepting and even appreciating your authentic autistic self instead of the masked, pseudo-neurotypical version you've presented to the world.

Many autistic women develop eating disorders partly because autism itself feels unacceptable. You've spent years trying to be normal, fit in, hide your differences. The exhaustion of constant masking plus the pain of rejection when your mask slips creates profound self-hatred. Eating disorders offer to perfect your body when your brain feels irreparably imperfect. If you could just lose enough weight, exercise enough, control yourself enough, maybe you'd finally be acceptable (Bargiela et al., 2016).

Recovery requires dismantling this belief system. Your autistic neurology isn't a flaw requiring compensation through body control. It's a neurological difference that affects how you process information, regulate emotions, experience sensory input, and interact socially. Some aspects create challenges. Some aspects create strengths. It's simply how your brain works.

Self-compassion practices for autistic identity:

Acknowledge masking costs: Recognize how much energy masking requires. You're not lazy or weak for finding social interaction exhausting. You're expending enormous effort appearing neurotypical in situations that don't accommodate your neurology. This effort is real and valid. You deserve rest and recovery from it.

Identify authentic preferences: Eating disorders often develop alongside losing track of authentic self. What do you actually enjoy vs. what you think you should enjoy? What genuinely interests you vs. what seems appropriate? Reconnecting with authentic preferences—special interests, comfortable activities, actual values—helps rebuild identity beyond eating disorder and masked autism.

Challenge ableist beliefs: You've internalized messages that autistic traits are wrong, childish, or broken. These are ableist beliefs, not truth. Stimming isn't childish—it's regulation. Need for routine isn't rigidity—it's nervous system support. Sensory sensitivities aren't oversensitivity—they're neurology. Question every belief you have about autism that frames it as inferior to neurotypicality. These beliefs fuel eating disorder behaviors by making you believe you need fixing (Cage & Troxell-Whitman, 2019).

Find autistic community: Connecting with other autistic individuals—online communities, local groups, autistic-run organizations—provides perspective that neurotypical-dominated spaces can't offer. You see people living full lives with autism. You realize you're not broken or alone. Community validates experiences and normalizes autism in ways that combat eating disorder beliefs about needing to perfect yourself into neurotypicality.

Celebrate autistic strengths: Autism isn't just challenges. Pattern recognition, attention to detail, ability to focus intensely on interests, honesty, systematic thinking, creativity from different perspective—these are real strengths. Eating disorders want you focused exclusively on what's "wrong" with you. Deliberately acknowledge what's right. What can your autistic brain do that serves you well? What do you appreciate about yourself?

Accept the both/and: You can simultaneously acknowledge autism creates challenges while refusing to view autism as fundamentally broken or inferior. Yes, interoception difficulties make eating harder. Yes, emotional regulation differences create vulnerabilities to mental health struggles. And yes, you're a complete person who deserves acceptance, appropriate support, and freedom from eating disorder control. Both realities exist simultaneously.

Elena, a 31-year-old autistic teacher, spent years hating her autism. She saw every autistic trait as evidence of fundamental brokenness requiring correction. Her eating disorder promised to perfect her—if she could just control her body enough, maybe she'd finally be acceptable despite her autistic brain. Recovery involved grieving this belief system. Elena joined an online autistic community and encountered people who celebrated rather than tolerated their autism. Slowly, she began questioning whether autism was really the problem. Maybe the problem was living in a world not designed for autistic neurology. She started stimming visibly at home, stopped forcing herself through overwhelming social situations, requested accommodations at work, and deliberately engaged with special interests guilt-free. These changes didn't cure her autism (nothing will—autism isn't an illness). But they dramatically reduced the shame and self-hatred that had fueled her eating disorder. She wasn't trying to perfect herself into something else anymore. She was trying to live well as herself.

7.8 What This Means for You

Emotional recovery for autistic women requires different strategies than standard eating disorder treatment offers. Alexithymia, meltdowns, shutdowns, emotional intensity, and difficulties with traditional emotion regulation approaches mean you need adapted tools.

Work with alexithymia instead of fighting it—use simplified emotion categories, physical sensation mapping, and contextual clues rather than demanding sophisticated emotion identification. Recognize how meltdowns and shutdowns interact with eating disorder behaviors, and develop protocols that break the cycle through adequate nutrition and stress reduction.

Process emotions through structure, movement, and special interests rather than exclusively through verbal reflection. Reclaim stimming as legitimate regulation instead of using eating disorders as substitute. Manage overwhelm through appropriate accommodations and demand reduction, not through restriction or other eating disorder behaviors.

Maintain enough routine to support emotional stability while building flexibility to prevent eating disorder rigidity. Most importantly, develop self-compassion for your authentic autistic self. Your autism isn't something requiring correction through body control. It's your neurology. Recovery means living well with that neurology, accommodations and all.

Chapter 8.0: Living in Recovery

Recovery isn't a destination where you arrive and everything's perfect forever. It's a way of living—eating consistently enough to fuel your life, managing challenges without turning to eating disorder behaviors, and building a life worth nourishing. For autistic women, recovery looks different than standard eating disorder treatment suggests. It includes accommodations for sensory processing, structure for interoception difficulties, routines for emotional stability, and acceptance of neurodivergent food relationships that don't match neurotypical eating patterns.

This final chapter brings everything together. You'll learn to define recovery on your own terms, advocate for the accommodations you need, build support systems that understand both your autism and your eating disorder history, and create sustainable strategies for long-term freedom from eating disorder control.

8.1 Defining Your Recovery

Standard eating disorder recovery looks like intuitive eating, flexible food choices, eating in all social situations comfortably, no food rules, spontaneous eating patterns, and body acceptance at any size. That's the goal most treatment programs work toward. It's also largely incompatible with autistic neurology.

Autistic recovery from eating disorders includes accommodations that standard recovery doesn't require (Tchanturia et al., 2020). This doesn't make it lesser recovery—it makes it autism-adapted recovery. Here's what that might include:

Structured eating vs intuitive eating: As discussed throughout this book, many autistic individuals need structured eating schedules because interoception doesn't provide reliable hunger signals. Your recovery might mean eating at consistent times daily based on external cues rather than waiting for hunger. This is recovery. It's sustainable, health-supporting eating that works with your neurology.

Limited food variety with adequate nutrition: You might recover eating 30 foods instead of 300. If those 30 foods cover your nutritional needs and you can eat them consistently, that's recovery. Your eating disorder wants you to eat less with more restriction. Recovery means eating enough with enough variety for health. The specific number of foods doesn't matter if adequacy is met.

Sensory accommodations: Recovery might mean always avoiding certain textures that trigger genuine sensory distress, preparing foods in specific ways, eating alone sometimes to reduce sensory demands, or maintaining environment conditions that make eating possible. These aren't eating disorder behaviors—they're autism accommodations (Kinnaird et al., 2019).

Routine maintenance: Your recovery includes enough routine to support consistent eating and emotional regulation. Standard recovery pushes complete flexibility. Autistic recovery includes graduated flexibility within maintained structure. You can eat in imperfect circumstances, but you maintain basic routines because they support your functioning.

Different social eating patterns: You might never enjoy eating in loud, crowded restaurants. You might always prefer eating alone or only with specific trusted people. You might need to adapt social eating situations more than neurotypical people do. This is acceptable. Recovery doesn't require matching neurotypical social eating patterns.

Partial interoception reliance: You might always use some external frameworks for eating—alarms, meal plans, portion guides—because your interoception remains partially impaired. This is fine. Recovery doesn't require perfect internal signal processing. It requires consistent adequate nutrition using whatever combination of internal and external signals works for you.

Think about what recovery means for you specifically. What does life look like when eating is no longer dictating your choices? What accommodations do you need to eat consistently without eating disorder control? What does food freedom mean for an autistic person, recognizing that "freedom" might include some structure?

Raj, a 35-year-old autistic engineer, initially resisted recovery because standard recovery looked impossible. Eating randomly throughout the day? Eating whatever, whenever? That wasn't sustainable for him. His breakthrough came when his dietitian said, "Recovery for you might include eating at 8 AM, noon, 3 PM, and 7 PM daily. Same general times. Rotation of foods you can manage. Enough flexibility to handle schedule variations occasionally. That's still recovery—it's just autism-adapted recovery." Suddenly recovery looked achievable. Five years later, Raj maintains this structure. He's not intuitive eating. He's not spontaneously flexible. But he's consistently nourished, no longer using restriction to manage life, and living fully. That's recovery.

8.2 Advocating for Accommodations

If you seek eating disorder treatment after reading this book, you'll likely encounter programs not designed for autistic individuals. You need to advocate for adaptations. Here's how.

Before entering treatment:

Request autism-informed care: Ask directly if the program has experience treating autistic individuals with eating disorders. Do they employ clinicians trained in autism? Have they adapted protocols for autistic patients? If the answer is vague or dismissive, that's information about whether this program can serve you well.

Share autism education: Provide your treatment team with resources about autism and eating disorders. The PEACE Pathway research, academic articles about the comorbidity, information about sensory processing and interoception. Don't assume they already know. Many eating disorder professionals have limited autism training (Kinnaird et al., 2017).

Establish accommodations from start: Document needed accommodations before treatment begins. Sensory needs (lighting, noise levels, private eating space if group dining is intolerable), routine needs (predictable schedules, advanced notification of changes), communication needs (written information vs verbal, clear expectations), social needs (reduced group therapy or individual therapy priority). Get these documented as treatment plan components, not optional extras.

During treatment:

Distinguish autism from eating disorder: When treatment staff interpret autism traits as eating disorder symptoms, correct this gently but firmly. "I need to eat at the same time daily because of poor interoception, not eating disorder rigidity." "I'm avoiding this food due to sensory texture issues, not fear of calories." "I'm withdrawing because I'm sensorially overwhelmed, not resisting treatment." You shouldn't have to constantly educate, but sometimes you do.

Request specific adaptations: Don't just say "I need accommodations." Specify. "I need noise-canceling headphones during meals because the dining room is overwhelming." "I need written summaries of therapy sessions because I process information better reading than hearing." "I need individual therapy instead of group therapy because group social demands exhaust me." Specific requests are harder to dismiss than vague ones.

Involve autism specialists: If your treatment team lacks autism expertise, ask if you can bring in consultation from autism specialists. Maybe an outside occupational therapist can assess sensory needs. Maybe an autism-specialized psychologist can provide staff training. Treatment teams often welcome expert consultation when they recognize their knowledge gaps.

After treatment:

Maintain autism accommodations: Don't abandon accommodations because treatment is over. They're not temporary supports—they're ongoing needs. Keep structured eating times, sensory-friendly environments, routine maintenance, whatever helps you function well and eat consistently.

Find ongoing autism-informed support: Seek therapists, dietitians, and support groups that understand both autism and eating disorders. This combination is rare but increasingly available. The Eating Disorders and Neurodivergence Special Interest Group and similar organizations maintain directories of autism-informed eating disorder professionals.

Chen, a 32-year-old autistic artist, entered residential treatment with extensive documentation of her autism needs. The program initially resisted accommodations—"Everyone eats in the dining room, no exceptions." Chen advocated persistently, eventually escalating to administrators with research documentation and threat of ADA complaint. Finally, accommodations were granted: permission to eat in a quiet space, written meal plans instead of verbal instructions, reduced group therapy with increased individual sessions. Other patients benefited too—Chen's advocacy led the program to implement broader accommodations that helped multiple neurodivergent patients. Advocacy is exhausting when you're already struggling. But sometimes it's necessary, and your advocacy might benefit others beyond yourself.

8.3 Building Understanding Support

You need people who understand both identities—autistic and eating disorder history. People who recognize why you need routine without assuming it's eating disorder rigidity. People who respect sensory needs without thinking you're being difficult. People who accept that your eating patterns might always look somewhat different.

Finding these people:

Autistic community: Other autistic individuals understand sensory issues, interoception difficulties, emotional regulation challenges, and need for routine. They might not personally have eating disorder experience, but they understand the autism parts of your experience. Online communities (#ActuallyAutistic spaces, autism forums) provide connection and validation.

Eating disorder community with caveats: Traditional eating disorder recovery communities can be supportive, but be cautious. Content focusing heavily on intuitive eating or body positivity might not translate well to autistic recovery. Look for neurodivergence-inclusive eating disorder spaces specifically. The Eating Disorders and Neurodivergence community creates space for non-standard recovery paths.

Individual relationships: Some people naturally understand complex intersections even without direct experience. They listen, believe you, adapt to your needs, and accept differences. These people are gold. Cultivate these relationships. Don't waste energy on people who invalidate either your autism or your recovery needs (Cage & Troxell-Whitman, 2019).

Professional support: Therapists, dietitians, and medical providers who are educated about both conditions provide crucial ongoing support. They don't expect neurotypical eating patterns. They adapt treatment to match your neurology. They understand that your recovery might look different and that's acceptable.

What to communicate to support people:

Your specific accommodations: Explain what you need and why. "I eat at set times because my hunger signals are unreliable, and if I wait for hunger, I skip meals." "I need advance notice about social eating because processing the logistics requires preparation." "I can only handle short social visits because masking exhausts me."

Specific explanations help people understand and accommodate appropriately.

Your triggers and vulnerabilities: Let trusted people know what situations or comments trigger eating disorder urges or autistic overwhelm. "Comments about my eating patterns are triggering." "Surprise changes to plans increase my anxiety significantly." "I need to leave social situations when I'm overwhelmed, and it's not personal." Clear communication prevents misunderstandings.

How they can help: Don't make people guess. "You can support me by respecting my eating schedule even if yours is different." "Please don't suggest I should just relax and eat whatever—I need structure." "Check in without being controlling—ask how I'm doing, don't police my eating."

Boundaries around food and body: Establish clear boundaries. "I don't discuss weight or body size." "I don't participate in diet talk." "Please don't comment on my food choices or amounts." Protect your recovery by limiting exposure to triggering conversations.

8.4 Social Eating Strategies

Social eating remains challenging even in recovery. The sensory demands, social expectations, unpredictability, and attention on eating create perfect conditions for autistic overwhelm. You can't avoid social eating forever, but you can make it more manageable.

Choose venues strategically: Suggest quiet restaurants, outdoor settings with less echo, times when venues are less crowded. You're not being difficult—you're managing sensory demands so you can actually eat. Friends who care will accommodate. Friends who don't weren't friends worth keeping anyway.

Eat beforehand if needed: If a social situation is too overwhelming for eating, eat before or after. Some autistic individuals bring their own food to events. Some eat a full meal before social events and then order something small to avoid questions. Some eat after everyone leaves. This isn't ideal, but it's better than not eating or triggering eating disorder behaviors trying to force eating in overwhelming circumstances.

Practice declining politely: "No thank you" is a complete sentence. You don't owe explanations about why you're not eating something, why you're leaving early, or why you prefer certain restaurants. Eating disorder recovery sometimes teaches you to override all food refusals. Autistic recovery recognizes some refusals are legitimate sensory or accommodation needs. Trust yourself to distinguish.

Limit duration: Social eating doesn't require three-hour dinners. Suggest coffee (shorter duration, fewer eating demands), brief lunch meetings, or joining only for part of the event. Shorter exposures reduce overwhelm and make social eating more sustainable.

Have exit strategies: Know you can leave if overwhelming. This reduces anxiety about committing to social eating. "I can't stay long, but I'd love to see you for an hour." "I might need to leave early if I'm overwhelmed." Permission to exit makes entry easier.

Isabella, a 28-year-old autistic accountant, developed a social eating strategy that worked for her life. When friends invited her to loud restaurants, she suggested quieter cafes instead. When extended family hosted overwhelming holiday meals, she ate beforehand and joined for dessert only. When work required lunch meetings, she chose familiar restaurants where she knew she could order acceptable foods without extensive menu processing. She stopped forcing herself through eating situations that were genuinely intolerable. Some people judged her for this. Most people adjusted. Her eating stayed stable, and her social connections improved because she wasn't always exhausted and dysregulated from forced eating situations. She defined social eating on her terms rather than trying to match neurotypical patterns.

8.5 Preventing Relapse

Life stress happens. Jobs, relationships, losses, changes, unexpected challenges. For anyone with eating disorder history, stress increases relapse risk. For autistic individuals, the same stressors that trigger eating disorder urges also trigger autistic overwhelm—meaning you're hit twice as hard.

Early warning signs:

Eating pattern changes: Missing meals occasionally becomes missing meals frequently. Portion sizes shrink. Safe foods list tightens. Time-based eating structure loosens (in harmful direction). These changes signal returning restriction before you consciously recognize it.

Increased rigidity: Rules that were flexible become rigid again. Accommodations that supported recovery become restrictions. You can't eat if timing is slightly off. Foods must be prepared exactly one way. This progression from structure to rigidity indicates eating disorder thinking returning.

Social withdrawal: Avoiding social eating situations more frequently, canceling plans, isolating. Some social withdrawal is appropriate autism accommodation. Increasing withdrawal that disrupts relationships and life participation signals problems.

Body focus intensification: Increased mirror checking, body criticism, comparing yourself to others, clothing discomfort focus. These cognitive patterns precede behavioral changes. Catching them early allows intervention before full relapse.

Emotional numbness: Returning to restricted eating to dull emotions. Feeling flat, disconnected, less engaged with life. This was restriction's appeal initially—it might tempt you again during difficult periods.

Prevention strategies:

Maintain structure even when life changes: Changes disrupt routine, which triggers both autistic stress and eating disorder vulnerability. When life changes, eating structure stays consistent. This becomes your anchor during chaos. Everything else might be unpredictable, but eating remains structured and adequate.

Increase support during high stress: Don't wait for crisis to seek help. When you anticipate or experience elevated stress, proactively increase therapy frequency, connect with support people, use additional accountability for eating. Prevention is easier than crisis intervention.

Return to basics: If you notice early warning signs, return to your most structured recovery approach. Time-based eating, meal plans, external accountability, increased self-monitoring. Don't assume you're "past" needing structure. Structure is recovery for autistic brains, not just early recovery training wheels.

Distinguish accommodation from restriction: Constantly evaluate: Does this behavior support adequate eating or restrict it? Does this routine help me function or limit me? Does this rule serve my autism or my eating disorder? Maintain this discernment throughout recovery.

Address autism overwhelm: Often, eating disorder urges return because autistic stress is unmanaged. If you notice urges increasing, assess your overall overwhelm. Do you need more sensory accommodations? More recovery time? Reduced demands? Better emotional regulation support? Addressing autism needs often reduces eating disorder vulnerability (Tchanturia et al., 2020).

Emergency protocol: Create a specific plan for high-risk situations. Write it down. "If I notice restriction returning, I will: (1) Contact therapist immediately, (2) Return to full meal plan structure, (3) Increase accountability with trusted person, (4) Reduce demands where possible, (5) Use crisis supports if needed." Having a protocol reduces panic and provides clear action steps.

8.6 Relationships and Eating Together

Dating, long-term partnerships, and intimate relationships add layers to eating and autism. You're managing your own eating, your autism needs, relationship dynamics, and potentially your partner's responses to both.

What partners need to understand:

Your eating patterns: Explain your recovery eating approach—structure, accommodations, why certain things matter. "I eat at set times because my hunger signals don't work well" or "I have limited foods I can eat due to sensory processing—this isn't pickiness or eating disorder restriction."

Autism and relationship: Help partners understand autistic differences in communication, emotional processing, sensory needs, and social capacity. Many relationship conflicts come from neurological differences misinterpreted as personal rejection or lack of care. Education prevents misunderstandings.

Support vs control: Partners need to support recovery without policing eating. Support looks like respecting meal schedules, accommodating food preferences, understanding social eating limitations. Control looks like monitoring amounts, commenting on food choices, or trying to "fix" eating patterns. Clarify the difference explicitly.

What you need to navigate:

Shared meals: Living with partners involves shared eating. This requires negotiation. Maybe you eat some meals together and others separately. Maybe you eat the same foods but at your set times rather than spontaneous times. Maybe you eat different foods at the same table. Find what works for both partners without compromising your recovery.

Social couple events: Partner events add social pressure to eat in challenging circumstances. Communicate needs. "I can attend but might need to leave early." "I'll eat before we go." "Let's choose a quieter restaurant option." Partners who respect these needs support your recovery.

Physical intimacy: Body image issues from eating disorder history affect intimacy. Autism affects physical touch preferences and sensory sensitivities. Both need addressing. Communicate openly about what feels comfortable, what boundaries you need, and how your partner can support you feeling safe in your body.

Long-term considerations: Some autistic women with eating disorder history choose partners who naturally accommodate differences. Others choose partners requiring more education. Neither is wrong. But relationships where partners fundamentally don't accept your autism or recovery needs won't work long-term. Choose partners who appreciate you as you are, accommodations and all.

Sofia, a 30-year-old autistic social worker, married someone who initially didn't understand either autism or eating disorder recovery. Early years involved conflict—he wanted spontaneous dinner outings, she needed structured eating times. He suggested she should "just try" foods she sensory-avoided, misunderstanding her limitations. Through couples therapy with an autism-informed therapist and extensive education, he learned. He now plans restaurant choices considering sensory environment. He respects her eating schedule as legitimate health need. He understands her social capacity limits aren't personal rejection. Their relationship works because he adapted and she advocated. But it required effort from both. Partners willing to learn and adapt make autism-ED recovery more sustainable. Partners who won't accept differences make recovery harder.

8.7 Your Recovery Toolkit

These are the specific strategies and tools that support long-term recovery for autistic women. Copy this list. Adapt it. Make it yours.

Daily structure: Time-based eating schedule (breakfast, lunch, snack, dinner times), routine morning and evening regulation activities, predictable self-care patterns, regular sleep schedule.

Sensory management: Noise-canceling headphones, fidget tools, weighted blanket, comfortable clothing, control over lighting and temperature, sensory-friendly eating environment, stim breaks throughout day.

Meal planning: Template-based meal plans (protein + starch + vegetable + fat), rotation of acceptable foods, batch prep when executive function allows, pre-portioned options when needed, visual meal planning tools if helpful.

Emotional regulation: Stimming as primary regulation, special interest engagement for calming, movement for emotion release, simplified emotion identification system, structured processing methods (journaling, talking with trusted person), meltdown and shutdown protocols.

Interoception support: Alarms and reminders for meal times, energy level monitoring as hunger proxy, eating log for pattern identification, external portion guides when fullness signals unclear, body scan practices if tolerable.

Cognitive flexibility: Graduated flexibility practice within structure, multiple scripts for varied situations, challenge restrictive rules systematically, maintain helpful structure, distinguish accommodation from restriction regularly.

Social support: Autism community connections, eating disorder recovery community (neurodivergence-aware), individual relationships with understanding people, professional support team (autism-informed therapist, dietitian, medical provider).

Crisis resources: Emergency protocol for eating disorder urges, therapist crisis contact, supportive friends who can help in crisis, crisis hotlines (NEDA hotline: 1-800-931-2237), return-to-basics structured eating plan, clear warning signs list.

Self-compassion practices: Regular acknowledgment of masking costs, connection with autistic identity and community, challenge ableist beliefs about autism, celebrate autistic strengths, accept authentic preferences and needs, affirm that autism-adapted recovery is legitimate recovery.

8.8 Celebrating Neurodivergent Food Relationships

Here's the truth eating disorder treatment often misses: your relationship with food as an autistic person will probably always be somewhat different from neurotypical relationships with food. That's okay. Different isn't disordered.

Neurotypical food relationship: spontaneous, flexible, intuitive, highly social, easy variety, automatic hunger and fullness regulation.

Autistic food relationship: more structured, contains accommodations, relies on some external cues, sometimes solitary, limited but adequate variety, uses cognitive support for eating signals.

Both are acceptable. Both can be healthy. Neurotypical isn't the only valid way to eat. You're not failing if your eating includes structure, routine, accommodations, and differences. You're succeeding if your eating adequately nourishes you and doesn't control your life.

Celebrate what works for you:

Your structured eating times that ensure consistent nutrition. Your rotation of safe foods that covers nutritional needs. Your sensory accommodations that make eating possible. Your routine that supports emotional stability. Your self-advocacy that gets you appropriate treatment. Your persistence through recovery when standard approaches didn't work. Your resilience through both autism challenges and eating disorder challenges simultaneously.

You've done something remarkably difficult. You've recovered from an eating disorder as an autistic person using adapted approaches in a treatment system not designed for you. You've created a food relationship that works with your neurology instead of fighting against it. You've learned to eat consistently despite interoception difficulties, sensory challenges, executive function limitations, and emotional regulation differences.

That's tremendous. Genuinely. Whether your recovery includes 20 foods or 200, whether you eat intuitively or on schedule, whether you eat socially or alone most of the time—you're feeding yourself adequately without eating disorder control. That's freedom. That's recovery. That's worth celebrating (Kinnaird et al., 2019).

Your autism isn't something you needed to overcome to recover. Your autism is part of you, and you recovered with accommodations and strategies that respect your neurology. The eating disorder was the problem. The autism is just your brain's operating system. It requires specific conditions to run well—structure, accommodations, support—but it's not broken. You're not broken. You're autistic, recovered from an eating disorder, and thriving in a way that works for your brain.

That's the goal. You've reached it. Now keep living it.

8.9 Taking It Forward

Recovery is ongoing. You don't graduate from needing accommodations, structure, or support. You integrate recovery principles into daily living and keep applying them. When stress increases, you return to basics. When life changes, you maintain eating structure. When autism overwhelm threatens to trigger eating disorder behaviors, you use your full toolkit of regulation strategies.

You advocate for accommodations in treatment, relationships, work, and life. You build support systems that understand both autism and eating disorder recovery. You define recovery on your terms rather than accepting neurotypical standards that don't fit your neurology. You maintain sensory-safe food relationships that prioritize adequacy over variety, structure over spontaneity, and self-acceptance over conformity.

Your recovery includes eating consistently with autism accommodations. It includes managing emotions without food control. It includes building a life worth nourishing. Most importantly, it includes accepting yourself—autistic traits, eating differences, accommodations, and all.

Living in recovery means choosing adequate nutrition even when life is hard. It means maintaining structure even when eating disorders promise relief through restriction. It means respecting your autism needs while refusing eating disorder control. It means thriving as the autistic person you are, fed adequately and free from eating disorder bondage.

You've learned the strategies. You have the tools. You understand your specific needs. Now you live it—one structured meal, one accommodation, one day at a time. That's recovery for autistic women. That's freedom. That's your life, reclaimed.

References

American Psychiatric Association. (2013). Diagnostic and statistical manual of mental disorders (5th ed.).

Antony, M. M., Ledley, D. R., & Heimberg, R. G. (Eds.). (2007). Improving outcomes and preventing relapse in cognitive-behavioral therapy. Guilford Press.

Babb, C., Brede, J., Jones, C. R. G., Serpell, L., Mandy, W., & Fox, J. (2021). 'It's not that they don't want to access the support... it's the impact of the autism': The experience of eating disorder services from the perspective of autistic women, parents and healthcare professionals. Autism, 25(5), 1409-1421.

Bargiela, S., Steward, R., & Mandy, W. (2016). The experiences of late-diagnosed women with autism spectrum conditions: An investigation of the female autism phenotype. Journal of Autism and Developmental Disorders, 46(10), 3281-3294.

Baron-Cohen, S. (1997). Mindblindness: An essay on autism and theory of mind. MIT Press.

Baron-Cohen, S. (2009). Autism: The empathizing-systemizing (E-S) theory. Annals of the New York Academy of Sciences, 1156(1), 68-80.

Bentz, M., Westwood, H., Jepsen, J. R., Plessen, K. J., & Tchanturia, K. (2017). The autism diagnostic observation schedule: Patterns in individuals with anorexia nervosa. European Eating Disorders Review, 25(6), 571-579.

Bird, G., & Cook, R. (2013). Mixed emotions: The contribution of alexithymia to the emotional symptoms of autism. Translational Psychiatry, 3(7), e285.

Brede, J., Babb, C., Jones, C., Elliott, M., Zanker, C., Tchanturia, K., Serpell, L., Fox, J., & Mandy, W. (2020). 'For me, the anorexia is just a symptom, and the cause is the autism': Investigating restrictive eating disorders in autistic women. Journal of Autism and Developmental Disorders, 50(12), 4280-4296.

Brosnan, M., Lewton, M., & Ashwin, C. (2016). Reasoning on the autism spectrum: A dual process theory account. Journal of Autism and Developmental Disorders, 46(6), 2115-2125.

Cage, E., & Troxell-Whitman, Z. (2019). Understanding the reasons, contexts and costs of camouflaging for autistic adults. Journal of Autism and Developmental Disorders, 49(5), 1899-1911.

Cermak, S. A., Curtin, C., & Bandini, L. G. (2010). Food selectivity and sensory sensitivity in children with autism spectrum disorders. Journal of the American Dietetic Association, 110(2), 238-246.

Dajani, D. R., & Uddin, L. Q. (2015). Demystifying cognitive flexibility: Implications for clinical and developmental neuroscience. Trends in Neurosciences, 38(9), 571-578.

Demetriou, E. A., Lampit, A., Quintana, D. S., Naismith, S. L., Song, Y. J. C., Pye, J. E., Hickie, I., & Guastella, A. J. (2018). Autism spectrum disorders: A meta-analysis of executive function. Molecular Psychiatry, 23(5), 1198-1204.

DuBois, D., Ameis, S. H., Lai, M. C., Casanova, M. F., & Desarkar, P. (2016). Interoception in autism spectrum disorder: A review. International Journal of Developmental Neuroscience, 52, 104-111.

Garfinkel, S. N., Seth, A. K., Barrett, A. B., Suzuki, K., & Critchley, H. D. (2015). Knowing your own heart: Distinguishing interoceptive accuracy from interoceptive awareness. Biological Psychology, 104, 65-74.

Garfinkel, S. N., Tiley, C., O'Keeffe, S., Harrison, N. A., Seth, A. K., & Critchley, H. D. (2016). Discrepancies between dimensions of interoception in autism: Implications for emotion and anxiety. Biological Psychology, 114, 117-126.

Grove, R., Hoekstra, R. A., Wierda, M., & Begeer, S. (2018). Special interests and subjective wellbeing in autistic adults. Autism Research, 11(5), 766-775.

Herbert, B. M., & Pollatos, O. (2012). The body in the mind: On the relationship between interoception and embodiment. Topics in Cognitive Science, 4(4), 692-704.

Hollocks, M. J., Lerh, J. W., Magiati, I., Meiser-Stedman, R., & Brugha, T. S. (2019). Anxiety and depression in adults with autism spectrum disorder: A systematic review and meta-analysis. Psychological Medicine, 49(4), 559-572.

Horner, K. M., Schubert, M. M., Desbrow, B., Byrne, N. M., & King, N. A. (2015). Acute exercise and gastric emptying: A meta-analysis and implications for appetite control. Sports Medicine, 45(5), 659-678.

Jenkinson, P. M., Taylor, L., & Laws, K. R. (2018). Self-reported interoceptive deficits in eating disorders: A meta-analysis of studies using the eating disorder inventory. Journal of Psychosomatic Research, 110, 38-45.

Kapp, S. K., Steward, R., Crane, L., Elliott, D., Elphick, C., Pellicano, E., & Russell, G. (2019). 'People should be allowed to do what they like': Autistic adults' views and experiences of stimming. Autism, 23(7), 1782-1792.

Kinnaird, E., Norton, C., & Tchanturia, K. (2017). Clinicians' views on working with anorexia nervosa and autism spectrum disorder comorbidity: A qualitative study. BMC Psychiatry, 17(1), 292.

Kinnaird, E., Stewart, C., & Tchanturia, K. (2019). Investigating alexithymia in autism: A systematic review and meta-analysis. European Psychiatry, 55, 80-89.

Kitayama, S., Markus, H. R., & Kurokawa, M. (2000). Culture, emotion, and well-being: Good feelings in Japan and the United States. Cognition & Emotion, 14(1), 93-124.

Loomes, R., Hull, L., & Mandy, W. P. L. (2017). What is the male-to-female ratio in autism spectrum disorder? A systematic review and meta-analysis. Journal of the American Academy of Child & Adolescent Psychiatry, 56(6), 466-474.

Lucarelli, J., Pappas, D., Welchons, L., & Augustyn, M. (2017). Autism spectrum disorder and avoidant/restrictive food intake disorder. Journal of Developmental and Behavioral Pediatrics, 38(1), 79-80.

Macht, M. (2008). How emotions affect eating: A five-way model. Appetite, 50(1), 1-11.

Mazefsky, C. A., Herrington, J., Siegel, M., Scarpa, A., Maddox, B. B., Scahill, L., & White, S. W. (2013). The role of emotion regulation in autism spectrum disorder. Journal of the American Academy of Child & Adolescent Psychiatry, 52(7), 679-688.

Mehling, W. E., Acree, M., Stewart, A., Silas, J., & Jones, A. (2018). The Multidimensional Assessment of Interoceptive Awareness, Version 2 (MAIA-2). PLoS ONE, 13(12), e0208034.

Nicely, T. A., Lane-Loney, S., Masciulli, E., Hollenbeak, C. S., & Ornstein, R. M. (2014). Prevalence and characteristics of avoidant/restrictive food intake disorder in a cohort of young patients in day treatment for eating disorders. Journal of Eating Disorders, 2, 21.

Parsons, M. A., Omata, W., Storer, A., & Hart, S. (2023). Autism diagnosis in females by eating disorder professionals. Journal of Eating Disorders, 11(1), 78.

Quattrocki, E., & Friston, K. (2014). Autism, oxytocin and interoception. Neuroscience & Biobehavioral Reviews, 47, 410-430.

Russell, J. (Ed.). (1997). Autism as an executive disorder. Oxford University Press.

Samson, A. C., Huber, O., & Gross, J. J. (2012). Emotion regulation in Asperger's syndrome and high-functioning autism. Emotion, 12(4), 659-665.

Tavassoli, T., Miller, L. J., Schoen, S. A., Nielsen, D. M., & Baron-Cohen, S. (2014). Sensory over-responsivity in adults with autism spectrum conditions. Autism, 18(4), 428-432.

Tchanturia, K., Dandil, Y., Li, Z., Smith, K., Leslie, M., & Byford, S. (2021). A novel approach for autism spectrum condition patients with eating disorders: Analysis of treatment cost-savings. European Eating Disorders Review, 29(3), 514-518.

Tchanturia, K., Smith, K., Glennon, D., & Burhouse, A. (2020). Towards an improved understanding of the anorexia nervosa and autism spectrum comorbidity: PEACE pathway implementation. Frontiers in Psychiatry, 11, 640.

Tomchek, S. D., & Dunn, W. (2007). Sensory processing in children with and without autism: A comparative study using the short sensory profile. American Journal of Occupational Therapy, 61(2), 190-200.

Westwood, H., Eisler, I., Mandy, W., Leppanen, J., Treasure, J., & Tchanturia, K. (2016). Using the Autism-Spectrum Quotient to measure autistic traits in anorexia nervosa: A systematic review and meta-analysis. Journal of Autism and Developmental Disorders, 46(3), 964-977.

Westwood, H., Mandy, W., & Tchanturia, K. (2017). Clinical evaluation of autistic symptoms in women with anorexia nervosa. Molecular Autism, 8, 12.

Westwood, H., & Tchanturia, K. (2017). Autism spectrum disorder in anorexia nervosa: An updated literature review. Current Psychiatry Reports, 19(7), 41.

www.ingramcontent.com/pod-product-compliance
Lightning Source LLC
LaVergne TN
LVHW022105200926
848481LV00003B/1067
9781923646230